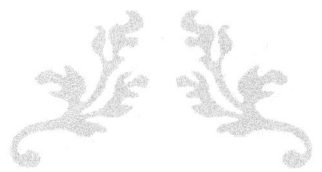

HOMEOPATHIC APPROACH FOR INJURIES

For students and beginners

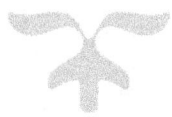

DR. SHEETAL SATAM
BHMS (MUMBAI), CCH (USA), MPH (USA)

Contents

Dedication

This book is dedicated to my loving husband, for his love, support, and encouragement throughout writing this book. Thank you so much for constantly encouraging me, without him I would have not been able to complete this book so soon.

Also special thanks to my father and mother-in-law and my parents for their endless support and encouragement.

Introduction to Homeopathy

Chapter 1: What is Homeopathy?

I. Introduction

Homeopathy is an art and system of medicine founded by German physician Dr. Samuel Christian Hahnemann in 19th century. *Homois* in Greek means 'similar' while *pathos* means 'suffering'. The original idea of homeopathy i.e 'like cures like' came from Hippocrates.[1] Over 2000 years ago, Hippocrates wrote about two different approaches towards healing:

1) Antipathic (Use of contrary medicines to restore the body to sick).
    Examples of Antipathic medicines – Use of anti-inflammatory to reduce the inflammation or administer laxative for constipation.

2) Homeopathic (Use of similar medicines that has caused the disease to restore the health). Example of Homeopathic medicines – Allium cepa is a common homeopathic remedy for hay fever, prepared from onion. When you peel or cut the onion a healthy person will start with runny nose, and watering from eyes, mild itching and burning in eyes. These symptoms are very similar to hay fever. Hence if a person is affected with hay fever like symptoms, Allium Cepa is a common remedy which restores the health of a person. It does not mean that Allium Cepa will cure all kind of hay fever, but it will only cure if the symptoms mimic an exposure to onion.

    Based on above homeopathic approaches, Hahnemann founded and elaborated this science. In eighteenth century he discovered that a medicine that could produce particular symptoms or a disease in a healthy living, would cure the same symptoms or disease when found in the sick.

i. Founder of Homeopathy

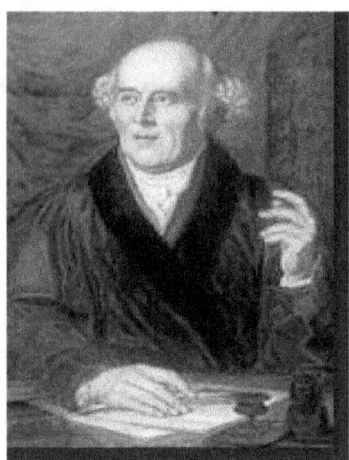

Dr. Samuel Hahnemann

Samuel Hahnemann (1755 – 1843) is a father of modern homeopathy. He studied medicine and completed his degree Doctor of Medicine in 1779. In 1780 he established his first practice, however it lasted for only 9 months. During his era, the therapies like bloodletting, purging and use of harsh drugs were the current therapies and were inhumane to Dr. Samuel Hahnemann's principles. He gave up his medical practice because he was dissatisfied with the way patients were treated at that time. According to him, modern medicine did not cure the sick, but increased the risk of injury. Since he had his wife and children to support he took on a work as a translator to supplement his income.

While translating a book "A Treatise of Materia Medica" by Dr. William Cullen, he came across the usefulness of Cinchona bark for treatment of Malaria due to it bitter and astringent properties. However Dr. Hahnemann believed this does not make sense that bitter and astringent properties helped to cure malaria as there are several other plants with similar properties but not useful in treating malaria. Hence he decided to conduct an experiment with Cinchona bark on himself. He began taking repeated does of this herb until his body responded to its toxic dose. His body produced symptoms similar to malaria (fever, chills, and fatigue). Hahnemann hypothesized that this remedy was useful for treating malaria because it has ability to produce the malaria like symptoms. From this experiment he derived the principle 'Like Cures Like' and also known as Law of Similars.

After this experiment, he began taking other herbs and started recording the symptoms. While doing these experiments he came up with an idea of 'minimum dose'. During the experiments he noticed that some of the substance were toxic and produced side-effects. Hence he started experimenting with small doses. To his surprise he noticed that the remedy actually worked better the more it is diluted. It means smaller doses worked better that larger doses. He made the smaller doses by repeatedly diluting and shaking (succession) each medicine to reduce its toxic effect. However Hahnemann was disliked because he recommended the use of single and small doses at a time.

ii. Criticism of Homeopathy

Orthodox medicine was threatened by Homeopathy because it offered systematic basis for its therapeutic practice. Many pharmaceutical companies disliked homeopathy because homeopathy can cure or reduce the suffering in systematic way using single, minimal dose, which is very cost-effective than conventional medicines.

The year 1812 – 1818 Hahnemann's practice flourished at Lipzig. However group orthodox physicians and pharmacists filed a case against Hahnemann to prevent him dispensing his own medicines. Unfortunately Hahnemann lost his case, closed his practice and moved to the city of Kothen in 1821.

He started his practice in Kothen with the permission from the city and settled there for 14 years. During these years he published his book named 'Chronic Diseases, Their Peculiar Nature, and Their Homeopathic Treatment.

In 1831, Asiatic Cholera Epidemic struck Europe. Hahnemann treated cholera using certain protocol, included sanitation, cleanliness, ventilation and disinfection, which helped to reduce the mortality to 20% which was 50% with conventional treatment. Hahnemann's article about treatment of cholera created criticism. His articles and his practice was banned again in Kothen.

II. Principles of Homeopathy

Like other system of medicine, Homeopathy is also based on certain principles. Principles basically means a rule, a law or the fact that explains how something works or something happens. Law means a rule of conduct or action formally recognized or established. These Homeopathic principles will guide you to understand and practice homeopathy in a right way. These fundamental principles are explained by Hahnemann in Organon of Medicine.

- Law of Similars
- Law of Simplex
- Law of Minimum
- Doctrine of Drug Proving
- Doctrine of Drug Dynamization
- Theory of Vital Force
- Theory of Chronic Disease

- 'Similia Similibus Curanter' or Law of Similars'

  First fundamental principle of homeopathic system is **'Similia Similibus Curanter' or Law of Similars' (Let like be cured by like).** This is the most important principle as homeopathy is based on this principle. This principle implies that a substance capable of producing a disease or disorder in a healthy person is also capable to treat the sick with similar symptoms.

  Dr. Hahnemann developed the Law of Similars and has stated in the aphorism 26 in the *Organon of Medicine* book, He states that "A weaker dynamic affection is permanently extinguished in the living organism by a stronger one, if the latter (whilst differing in kind) is very similar to the former in its manifestations." [2] It means the disease is rapidly and permanently cured if the symptoms of the chosen medicine are similar to the disease symptoms but superior in strength.

  1) An example of Allium Cepa demonstrates the law of similar. The above examples of allium cepa concludes that what onion can produce in the healthy state, it will treat in the sick. Let me give you one more example to better understand this principle.

  2) Consider a healthy person who consumes a cup of strong coffee will experience certain symptoms like insomnia, restlessness, palpitation, excited and hyperactive, hence we usually do not take coffee at night. In healthy person coffee produces these symptoms and hence it should be able to relieve the similar symptoms in the sick. A homeopathic remedy called as Coffea Cruda, prepared from Coffee would relieve the similar symptoms.

  Many conventional medicine use homeopathy like treatment which are based on Law of Similars. For instance, digitalis is used in treatment of heart conditions. Digitalis if taken in healthy state produces the similar heart conditions. Another example is immunization. Immunizations are based on Law of Similars. A small dose of vaccine provides protection from similar kind of diseases. For instance, Polio vaccine protects the healthy subjects from Polio disease.

  Law of Similars helps to heal the body, and makes the body capable to fight against the disease on its own.

- Law of Simplex (The single remedy)

  Homeopathy is based on another important principle - **Law of Simplex (The single remedy).** According to Dr. Hahnemann, one single remedy should be administered at a time because only one remedy can be the exact similar to the presenting disease at a time. Additionally, during the drug proving, drugs are proved singly and hence the effect of more than one remedy is not known. Suppose if a homeopath prescribe mixture of 2-3 remedies at a time, one of the might act very well but he will not know which remedy has acted on the patients. Also prescription of more than one remedy can cause adverse effects on the body.

- Law of Minimum (Minimum Dose)

Once a homeopathic remedy is selected, selection of proper dose is important too. Law of Minimum states that a medicine should be given in minute or minimum dose. Minute or minimum dose means the smallest quantity of medicine that produces excitation of vital force which is sufficient to produce necessary changes and remedial effect. If the medicine is selected based on the totality of symptoms then minimum amount of medicine is required to restore the sick to healthy.

Some of the physicist and scientist have observed and believed in this principle. **Arndt-Schultz law** which states that *'For every substance, small doses stimulate, moderate doses inhibit, large doses kill.'* [3] In other words, the same substance can cure a person in smaller dose or can have opposite action if given in the larger doses. Hence we can say that the same remedy can cure a patient or produce the toxic drug effect.

Even a French mathematician, **Maupertius**, also observed this same principle and stated, *'The quantity of action necessary to affect any change in the nature is the least possible, an infinitesimal'.* [4] Similarly, the minimum dose is a requirement for a complete cure.

There are several advantages of prescribing minimum dose:

1. Avoids unwanted aggravation
2. The smallest dose does not cause any organic damage and thus no drug effect or side effects of the medicine

- Doctrine of Drug Proving

Drug is any material agent, ingestion of which is capable of disturbing the balances of vital force. Drug proving is the systematic process of evaluation of the disease producing power of drug or substance on the healthy human beings of different sexes, age groups and different places. In simple terms, drug proving means the healthy human volunteers take a medicine for experimental purpose and note the changes produced in his / her functions which is expressed in the form of mental and physical symptoms.

Dr. Hahnemann developed the drug proving and described the appropriate method of drug proving in 'Organon of Medicine'. In drug proving, appropriate medicine in various potency is administered to a group of healthy human beings. The volunteers are instructed to take the medicine until they develop the symptoms; carefully observe and note down each and every symptoms, feelings, sensations or any deviation from the normal functioning of the body parts and organs.[2]

Once the proving is done, the symptoms reported by the provers are assessed and evaluated carefully and the result of this work is compiled in the book 'Materia Medica Pura'. This proved drug can be administered to as a curative remedy to the sick when he presents the similar group of symptoms as the healthy provers produced during drug proving. Usually the well proved drugs are prescribed to the patients.

To conduct the drug proving it is mandatory to choose the healthy human beings because if the diseased or sick individual is chosen, his disease symptoms will merge with the new proved symptoms. Hence it will be difficult to get the accurate picture of a drug or remedy.[2]

Drug proving is only done on human beings because they can describe the physical and emotional sensations and feelings precisely. Humans can record the subjective symptoms, and any subtle deviation in the normal functioning. Animals do not give subjective or mental symptoms. It is merely impossible to get the finer symptoms and modalities in animal provings. The effects of same drug is different in animals and humans.[2]

- Doctrine of Drug Dynamism

  To achieve the maximum benefit of the drug, it must be administered in the dynamic form because the dynamic quality of the drug that affects the vital force and not the physical and chemical properties of the drug.

Drug is usually in the material or crude form, it has to act on dynamic level of human being. In order to do this, Hahnemann began the experiment with the application of proven drugs on the sick where he used the proven drugs in full strength but he observed aggravation in the patients. After careful observation, he started diluting the drug, to his surprise he noticed better curative power in the diluted drugs than the drugs with full strength. Following this experiment he came up with the 'Principle of Potentisation'. The concept of potentisation is explained in detail in the following chapter. Hence the drug dynamism is also known as potentisation, where the drug is diluted to such a smaller quantity that it losses it's physical and chemical properties and only left with dynamic properties. Thus in diseased person the medicine acts on the plane same as the plane on which life force or vital force works.

There are several advantages of drug dynamisn or potentisation. They are as follows:

Firstly, the action of the potentised medicines is deeper, longer and curative. Secondly, the medicinal power increases dynamically by the process of potentisation, hence such medicines able to stimulate the defective vital force and restore the sick to a healthy state. Also the toxic materials like poisons and venoms when potentised are rendered harmless and can be used as therapeutic agents to cure the sick. Finally the aggravation from the potentised medicine is minimized because the process of potentisation reduce the quantity of medicinal substance and enhance the quality of substance.

- Theory of Vital Force

All living organism are regulated by Vital force. Vital force is an invisible force which activate the organism. It is the most integral part of any organism. Vital force performs all functions, and regulate the sensations of the human body. No vital force means no regulation of sensations and loss of functions of the body. Hence vital force is the most essential part of living being.[2] Vital force have been given different names in different culture and societies. It is also called as *life energy, vital energy, life principle and life force*. Dr. Hahnemann called it as *'Vital Force'*. Hence we will call it as vital force.

When a person falls sick, it is this vital force that is deranged. This vital force produces signs and symptoms like headache, fever, cold, cough, etc. However these symptoms are secondary changes which are the products of deeper disturbances, mainly mental, emotional or psychic disturbances. This disturbance in vital force is caused by mental sufferings like mental stress, anxiety, shock, deep longstanding grief, disappointment, etc.

Remember it is a vital force that is deranged to such an abnormal state, that can furnish the organism and thus disease settles in. Hence in disease, there is dynamic derangement of the vital force, which leads to disharmony and alteration of all the bodily functions and sensations.[2]

Dr. Hahnemann has described the concept of vital force in the Organon of Medicine in the aphorism 9 and 10:[2]

Aphorism 9: *In the healthy condition of man, the spiritual vital force (autocracy), the dynamis that animates the material body (organism), rules with unbounded sway, and retains all the parts of the organism in admirable, harmonious, vital operation, as regards both sensations and functions, so that our indwelling, reason-gifted mind can freely employ this living, healthy instrument for the higher purposes of our existence.*

Aphorism 10: *The material organism, without the vital force, is capable of no sensation, no function, no self preservation; it derives all sensation and performs all the functions of life solely by means of the immaterial being (the vital principle) which animates the material organism in health and in disease.*

In further aphorisms dr. Hahnemann has explained the dynamic cause of disease of all disease. I recommend all of you to read, and understand these aphorism in order to understand the basic concept of vital force.

- Theory of Chronic Disease

Dr. Hahnemann observed during his homeopathy practice that the diseases used to respond well after administering the similimum remedy however the disease used to come back after certain period of time. In acute cases he noticed that remedy responded well with no relapses but in chronic cases the disease relapses. After 12 years of careful study and observation, he came to a conclusion that some obstacle still exists in spite of all corrective measures. He discovered that these obstacles are disease producing agents, which are dynamic in nature. He named them as 'Chronic Miasms'. He classified miasms into three category - Psora, Sycosis and Syphilis.

Let me explain you these miasms in brief here.

Psora - Hahnemann called Psora as the mother of all chronic diseases and almost 80% of chronic diseases fall into this category. Psora is an internal disease, persists throughout the life, unless it is cured. It represents externally as itch or local skin disease, however it is a manifestation of an internal disorder. It should never be treated by external remedies. Diseases like psoriasis, eczema is included in this category.[6]

Sycosis – Hahnemann observed the sycosis is caused by suppressed gonorrhea and passed to few generations. Mainly it is caused by a primary infection which is non-heritant in nature, suppressed by allopathic medications. Sycosis is denoted by over functioning or over production of ailments. Sycosis produces infiltrations, indurations, and over growth.[6] The diseases like cancer, rheumatism, asthma, are sycotic in nature.

Syphilis – Syphilitic miasm is acquired primarily by heredity. The syphilitic miasm creates the predisposition to illnesses that reflect the deeper nature of syphilis without necessarily representing its common presentation. This miasm is responsible for nervous, and psychological disorders like suicidal impulses, depression, insanity, etc. [6]

Miasm is very important topic for homeopathic professionals especially for beginner to understand the theory and philosophy first before going for practical application. The practical application of miasm is not very easy and it may confuse the beginners. So I would recommend to initially understand the basic concept of the miasms.

III.   Conclusion

- Homeopathy is an art and system based on the principle of 'Like cures like' which means a substance that could produce particular set of symptoms or a disease in a healthy living, would cure the same symptoms or disease when found in the sick. This principle was originally discovered by Hippocrates 2000 years back.

- Dr. Samuel Hahnemann, elaborated the Hippocrates approach and founded homeopathy.

- Even though Hahnemann's practice of homeopathy flourished in 18th century, orthodox medicine always criticized his work and threatened homeopathy.

- Dr. Hahnemann translated and published several books, some of them were 'Materia Medica Pura', 'Chronic Diseases, Their Peculiar Nature, and Their Homeopathic Treatment'.

- Dr. Hahnemann laid down 7 fundamental principles in homeopathy. These principles guide and direct every practitioner towards the cure.

IV.   References

1. Lockie, D. A. (2000). *Encyclopedia of Homeopathy.* USA: DK Publishing Inc.

2. Hahnemann, S. *Organon of Medicine, 6th Edition*

3. *Arndt–Schulz rule*. Retrieved from Wikipedia:
       http://en.wikipedia.org/wiki/Arndt%E2%80%93Schulz_rule

4. *Pierre Louis Maupertuis*. Retrieved from Wikipedia:
       http://en.wikipedia.org/wiki/Pierre_Louis_Maupertuis#Least_Action_Principle

5. Roberts, H. A. (n.d.). *Principles and art of cure by homeopathy.* B. Jain Publisher Pvt Ltd.

6. Morrell, P. (n.d.). *Hahnemann's miasm theory and miasm remedies* . Retrieved from Homeoint:
       http://homeoint.org/morrell/articles/pm_miasm.htm

Chapter 2: Selection of Remedy

I.   Introduction

Homeopathy do not treat the diseases, but it treats the diseased individual because it is a man who is diseased. Symptoms are present at the level of tissues and organs but the external manifestation of the symptoms are due to disturbances of vital force or energy. Hence it is essential to understand an individual in the disease and the disease in an individual which can be done by detail study of both the disease and the individual. Hence it is very important to determine the characteristics symptoms of the individual in order to select the proper remedy. Individualization play important role in remedy selection. If a practitioner fails to individualize a case he fails to restore the sick into healthy state. Let's understand in brief the meaning of individualization.

II.   Individualization

No two humans will have same physical, mental or emotional problems or even same disease. Even though diagnosis is the same, every individual will act and react to their sufferings in different manner. Here the process of individualization comes in to play. In order to treat a patient in a holistic way, homeopath try to find the unique characteristics in every individual that differentiate one person from another. And based on these unique characteristics homeopathic remedy is prescribed.

Basically, individualization is a method of determining the most striking, singular, uncommon and peculiar symptoms in a diseased individual. Individualization is a process that differentiate the physical, mental and emotional aspect of one person from another. Hence it deals with the process to distinguish, to discriminate, to differentiate, to particularize and to characterize an individual.

Let's take a simple example of seasonal flu, where common flu symptoms are running nose, sneezing, bodyache, headache, fever low or high grade, nose block and sometimes nausea. These are the common symptoms of flu. Although these symptoms direct towards the diagnosis of a disease (Flu), it does not direct a homeopath towards a remedy. In such case every homeopath is looking for unique or peculiar symptoms in their patients in order to prescribe the similimum remedy.

Along with these common symptoms if a patient complains of high grade fever with bodyache but still feels very active. Thirst is increased during the fever and appetite is perfectly normal. This becomes characteristic symptoms because very less number of patients would feel active with normal appetite during high grade fever. This kind of case taking helps to individualize a patient and stabilize them with perfect similimum remedy.

Individualization is usually obtained through two steps:

- Detail case taking: Case taking is a unique art of careful observation, conversation and collecting information from patients and their family members (attendees) through various ways like physical and clinical examination, history-taking, and observation. It includes noting of all the alterations produced during the diseased state in an individual. The practitioner must note down what the patient says in his/her own language. Practitioner must observe and note down the patients gestures, facial expressions and tone in order to get better understanding of the case. In acute cases, practitioner must note down the alterations produced during the acute stage of the illness. Detailed case taking helps to find a remedy for a patient through our knowledge of Materia Medica, Organon of Medicine ad Repertory.
Case taking is itself a vast topic to discuss and beyond limitation of this book. However case taking is explained in detail in Organon of Medicine and I would recommend to read it for further knowledge on case taking.

Following are the further details of the case which bring about individualization:
i. Details regarding evolution of the symptoms in terms of onset or pattern of symptoms (sudden or gradual onset, or an order of appearance of symptoms). Evolution of symptoms are important for individualization of the case. The study of evolution involves understanding of patient from birth, adolescence, phase of puberty, and adulthood. The study of evolution means adaptation of the patient in all these phases of life. Practitioner must understand clearly how the patient adapt himself during the particular major event in his life. Understanding of this adaptation helps to individualize the patient

    Example: Sudden onset of symptoms – Belladonna, Aconite
    Gradual or slow onset – Calcarea group

ii. Details regarding pathology of the disease (type of discharge)
    Example: Yellow to green discharge – Pulsatilla
    Watery arid discharge – Allium cepa

iii. Details regarding the cause of disease or ailments of the disease (emotional or mental cause)
    Example: Shock or grief – Ignatia
    Disappointment in love – Natrum Muriaticum

iv.　Details regarding characteristics of the symptoms (location, sensation, aggravation, amelioration, and concomitants).
Example: Time aggravation 4-8pm – Lycopodium
　　　　Joint pain better by continuous motion – Rhus tox.

v.　Details regarding socio-cultural background
Example: Rich and high class living with frequent indulgence with alcohol – Most likely Nux vomica

The above are individualizing symptoms applicable mainly in a chronic cases. However practitioner should not get biased based on the above remedies related to the symptoms. Overall case should be taken into consideration in order to prescribe a correct similimum remedy.

- Detail case analysis (processing): It is process of classification of symptoms which represents the characteristics and individualistic response. It involves the analysis of the characteristic and individualistic symptoms of the patients. During this process, repertory can be useful to come up with the group of remedies. However further materia medica references help to compare closely the group of remedies.
During this process the characteristic symptoms are subjected to gradation also called as 'evaluation of symptoms'. The high grade symptoms are repertorized to get the final remedy. Most of the time group of remedies come up after repertorization. With the help of materia medica knowledge, the practitioner select the final remedy for the group.
Thus this whole process helps in selection of similimum remedy.

III.　Conclusion

- Individualization is the only way to select the homeopathic remedy

- Individualization is the process of determining the most striking, singular, uncommon and peculiar symptoms in a diseased individual and differentiate the physical, mental and emotional aspect of one person from another.

- Case taking and case analysis are the two ways of individualizing a case or patient

- The knowledge of repertory and material medica is very important as they both help in determining the group of remedies.

- The knowledge of material medica helps to select the final homeopathic remedy.

Chapter 3: Dosage and Potency

I. Introduction

The holistic approach of homeopathy is based on correct dosage and potency. Dosage and potency are two different terms. Many beginners and students are confused with these terms. In homeopathy, dose means quantity, or repetition of a remedy. Potency means the strength of the homeopathic remedy. For instance, Arnica 200C 4 pills three times a day. Here *200C* is a potency of Arnica, it determines the strength of the remedy, while *three times a day* is the dose of this remedy. Dose is the 4 pellets, twice a day. While potencies are 30c, 200c, 1M, etc. Potency is the potentised homeopathic remedy prepared in three different scales and useful for prescribing purposes.

II. Potentisation and Scales of Potency

Potentisation is a systematic and scientific process of successively diluting a substance that remove the presence of actual physical substance however only dynamic substance is left behind. This process minimizes the toxic effects of the crude substance and maximizes the dynamic healing properties of the substance.

There are three different scale of potency. They are as follows:

- The Centesimal Scale
  This is the first scale of potentization that Dr. Hahnemann developed. It is denoted by a numerical designation of potency, followed by the suffix C. For example, 30C, 200C are belong to the centesimal scale. Here 'C' stands for Roman letter 100. Hence the centesimal scale is prepared with 1:100 dilution ratio. In simple words, one part of medicinal substance is diluted with 99 parts of water and alcohol and succussed for 10 times to make it 1C potency. Similarly, 2C can be prepared using one part of 1C potency (previous potency) and 99 parts of water and alcohol. Thus 3C, 4C.......30C...200C....1M... can be prepared. The Roman number 'M' here indicates that it is diluted and succussed 1000 times. Most of the practitioners commonly use

30C, 200C and 1M potency in their practice. 30C and lower is considered as lower potency, 200C, 1M and higher are considered as higher potency.

The homeopathic remedy in the centesimal scale is usually prepared by two method - Succussion and Trituration method

Succussion Method:
Succussion is a process of potentisation, by which preparation of medicine takes place by the use of a liquid vehicle like alcohol or water, by vigorously shaking the solution in definite method.
Succussion for the Centesimal scale:
First take a clean, glass phial. Take one part of medicinal substance and add 99 parts of water or alcohol. Make sure at least 1/3rd of phial remains empty. Then firmly cover the phial with a cork and shake it. Follow the directions to shake the phial. Grasp the phial in right hand with a thumb firmly over the cork and strike it with 10 powerful strokes of arm on left palm of your hand. Make sure each stroke ends with a jerk. After 10 stokes, it becomes 1C potency. In order to make successive potencies, mix one part of previous potency with 99 parts of water or alcohol. [7]

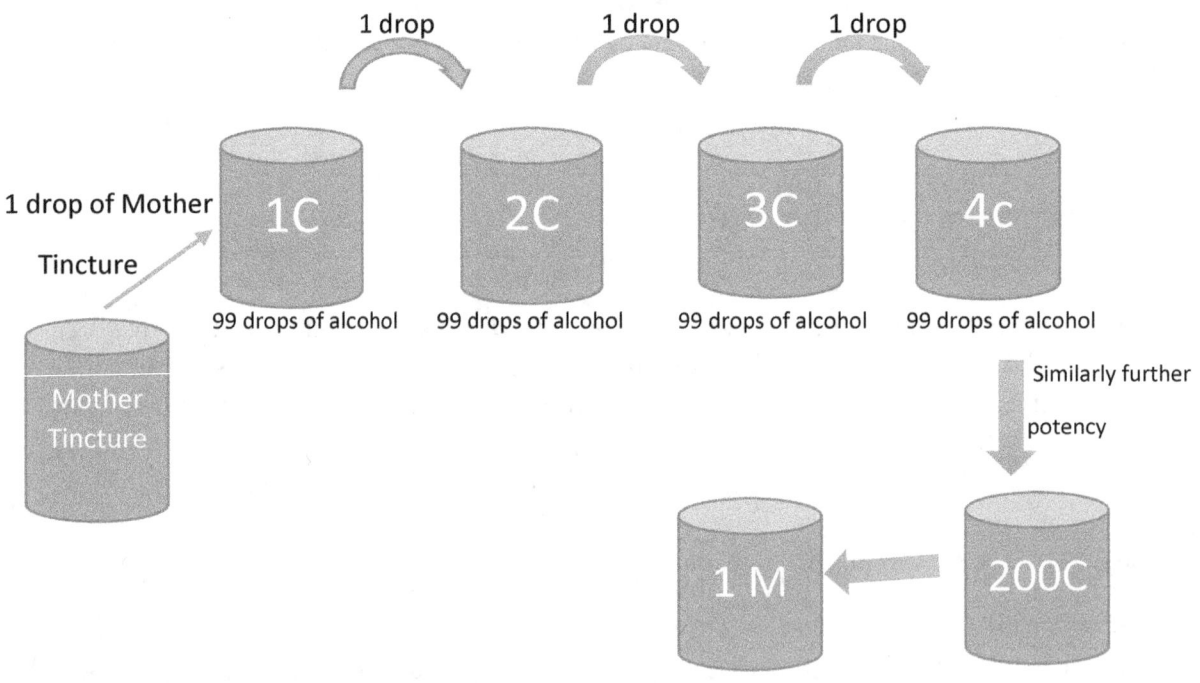

Preparation of the centesimal scale potency by succussion method

Trituration Method:

Trituration is a process of potentisation, by which preparation of medicine takes place by the use of a solid vehicle like sugar of milk, by grinding in definite order.

Trituration for the Centesimal scale:

One part by weight of the drug or medicinal substance is taken in a clean and unglazed porcelain mortar. 99 parts by weight of the sugar of milk is taken and divided in the ratio of 11:33:55 parts of sugar of milk.

One part of the drug and first part of sugar of milk is added in the mortar. The mixture is triturated for 20 minutes. Trituration is done using pestle to grind the mixture (added in the mortar) in anticlockwise or in circular fashion. Then mixture is scraped from the wall of mortar and mixed uniformly with the mixture.

In next stage the second part of sugar of milk (33 parts) is added in the same mortar and continue grinding, scraping and mixing for another 20 minutes in total.

In final stage, 55 parts of the sugar of milk is added in the same mortar for trituration. Thus trituration is carried out with three parts of sugar of milk. This gives 1C potency.

To achieve the 2C potency, 1 part of 1C potency is triturated for 60 minutes with 99 parts of sugar of milk.

In the similar manner further potency can be prepared.

Application and Use of the Centesimal scale

1. The Centesimal scale can be prescribed in liquid form or in tablets
2. The Centesimal scale is mainly useful to make higher potencies
3. The higher potencies are useful to treat deep seated chronic diseases.

- The Decimal Scale

  It is based on the principle that first potency should contain one-tenth of the original drug. This potency was first introduced by Dr. Constantine Herring. The decimal scale is denoted by suffixing the letter X. For instance, the first potency is 1X, second is 2X, 3X, 4X and so on..... 'X' stands for 10 in Roman letter. Hence the decimal scale potency is prepared with 1:10 dilution ratio, where one part of medicinal substance is mixed with 9 parts of water or alcohol. The preparation is same as the centesimal scale is, only difference is the use of 9 parts of water or alcohol instead of 99 parts.

The following is the succussion method for preparation of homeopathic remedy in the decimal scale:

In a clean glass phial, add 1 part of medicinal substance and 9 parts of alcohol and water, keep one-third of the phial empty for succussion. Close the cork of the phial tightly and perform succussion by firmly stroking the phial 10 times against the hard and elastic material. This becomes the first potency – 1X. To make the following potency, mix 1 drop of previous potency with 9 drops of alcohol or water. This becomes 2X potency. Thus in a similar way further potencies can be prepared.

The trituration method for preparation of homeopathic remedy in the decimal scale is same as the method of preparation in the centesimal scale. However instead of 99 parts of drug or medicinal substance, 9 parts of the drug or medicinal substance is used in the decimal scale. The process of trituration remains the same for the decimal scale.

Application and Use of the Decimal Scale

1. The Decimal scale potency is mainly useful to make lower potencies (up to 6X)
2. Decimal potency remedies are usually called as 'low potency' remedies, has less risk of producing proving symptoms, hence they can be repeated frequently.
3. These potencies are used in practice to a lower extent as they have limited use in curing the deep seated chronic diseases.
4. Decimal scale potencies are less effective than the centesimal scale potencies.

- 50 - Millesimal scale / Q Potency / LM Potency

This is the third scale of potency developed by Dr. Hahnemann. The potencies prepared according to 50 millesimal scale are denoted by prefixing '0'. It is also symbolically represented by the letter LM. This potency is represented in different ways. Following are some example:

0/1, 0/2, 0/3, 0/4, ...0/30

LM1, LM2, LM3, LM4, ... LM/30

Q1, Q2, Q3, ... Q30

LM is an abbreviated term given by Rudolf Flury. 'L' stands for Roman '50' while 'M' stands for Roman '1000'. It means this scale represents a serial dilution of 1:50,000 with each subsequent potency.[8]

The method of preparation of LM potency is quite different than the Centesimal and the Decimal potencies. Dr. Hahnemann described the method of preparation of LM potency in the footnote to the aphorism 270 in the 6th edition of Organon. Following is the method of preparation. [7,8]

- Prepare the three successive trituration (1C, 2C and 3C) from the medicinal substance. Here the ratio of each potency will be 1:100 since we are preparing with the centesimal scale.
- Take 1 grain of 3C and dissolve it is 500 drops of solution, having 100 drops of alcohol and 400 drops of distilled water. Here the ratio is 1:500.
- One drop of this solution is to be mixed with 100 drops of alcohol. This solution to be succussed for 100 times. This becomes the first potency of 50 millesimal scale (LM1 or 0/1). The proportion is 1:50,000 (1: 500 x 1: 100 = 1: 50,000).
- Soak 500 globules of same size in one drop of the first potency. Take one globule out of 500 and dissolve it in one drop of purified water. Add 100 drops of alcohol to it and success 100 times. This becomes second potency (LM2 or 0/2).
- In the similar way further potencies can be prepared.

Application and Use of the 50 Millesimal scale / LM potency

1. Fear of aggravation is low and medicine can be repeated frequently. However unnecessary repetition can cause proving of the remedy.
2. It has quick and rapid action.
3. 50 millesimal remedies are not dispensed in tablet forms. It should be given in liquid form because it becomes easier for homeopath to adjust the degree of dilution and number of succussions before each dose.
4. As the degree of dilution and number of succussions increase, greater is the effect of a remedy

You might have noticed that succession is the main part of the preparation of all the three scales. Succussion is basically a process of potentisation, by which preparation of medicine takes place by the use of a liquid vehicle like alcohol or water, by shaking in a definite method.

Many beginners ponder why succussion is required? Why not just dilute the medicinal substance or mother tincture and get the same potency? The answer is just diluting the medicine with alcohol or water was ineffective in treating the disease as per Dr. Hahnemann's observation. Succussion method requires mechanical energy which is delivered into the medicinal substance with violent jerks or strokes. Succussion of 10 strokes (centesimal and decimal scale) or 100 strokes (50 Milliesimal scale) adds kinetic energy to the substance. The repeated succussion of the remedy boost the therapeutic effect of the medicinal substance into the mixture of water and alcohol. Not even single molecule of the original substance remains at 12C or 24X potency and hence that remedy has no remains of toxic effects beyond these potencies. Hence we call homeopathy as free of side effects.

III.   Selection of Potency

The selection of potency and dose completely depends on the practicing homeopath. Generally any curable disease can be cured by any potency unless the selected remedy is the most homeopathic remedy. However the speed with which the cure will be affected depends on the potency of the drug. Hence we need to understand and select proper potency. [9]

Following are the considerations for choosing the potency of any homeopathic drug:[9]

- If the disease has strong pathology where the patient is deteriorating, prescribe lower potency medicines. Here we use lower potency because of the diminished vital force. In contrast if there are functional changes, without much gross involvement of the pathology, you can prescribe higher potency.
  For instance, in conditions like cholera, carcinoma, severe lower respiratory tract infection, etc. lower potency should be given.
  In conditions like seasonal flu, allergic rhinitis, anxiety, depression, etc., higher potency can be given.

- If the case demonstrates well defined symptoms, clear mental and physical picture of the patient and if a homeopath is completely sure about the remedy, then the higher potencies can be given (200 C and above or LM potency). In contrast, other than few prominent symptoms, the complete picture of the patient does not fit the remedy well, and if a homeopath is less sure about the remedy of choice, then go for the lower potencies like 12X, 30C, etc. The lower potency will produce less aggravation than the higher potency in case it is prescribed incorrectly.

- In chronic cases where the patients have used too many allopathic medicines, it is advisable to start with low or moderate potencies. Such patients usually have low susceptibility because of using too many allopathic medicines.

- Higher potencies are usually given to the patients who are quick to act and react, intelligent, and impulsive, while lower potencies are given who are mentally dull and sluggish, slow to act and react.

IV.   Selection of Dose

The selection of dose is basically means the either to prescribe single dose or repeat the remedy. Once the potency is selected, it dose selection depends on some of the following criteria's. [9]

- The high potency usually favors the single dose, although two or more doses of high potency may be given at short intervals, that is every 4, 6, 8, 12 or 24 hours especially in acute cases like fever.
- Lower potency remedies may be repeated frequently.
- If the selected remedy perfectly matches the mental and physical symptoms of the patient, then higher potency (200C and above) can be prescribed. Start with 200C potency, wait and watch the action of remedy, if requires, gradually increase the potency to 1M, 10M, etc. until the cure completes.
- Never repeat a remedy either is same potency or higher potency when patient himself is improving.
- Never change a remedy when symptoms are following the Hering's Law of Cure.
- You can repeat the single dose in same potency or higher potency if the patient complains of that his general sense of well-being has come to a standstill.

V.   Conclusion

- The understanding of the three scales of potentisation is very important for practical use.

- The Centesimal, Decimal and 50-Millisemal Scales are the three scales of potentisation.

- Succussion and trituration are the two methods of preparation of homeopathic remedies in above mentioned scales.

- Higher potency remedies act more deeply than lower potency remedies and the positive effect of the higher potency remedy remains for longer time than lower potency.

- Selection of correct remedy is critical for complete cure of the sick than correct selection of potency. Correct potency may enhance or change the therapeutic effect of the drug or remedy. Whatever potency is selected, if the remedy selected is correct it will lead to some improvement.

- On other hand, incorrect remedy will be of no value, whatever the potency prescribed. Hence selection of remedy is prime important than selection of dose or potency.

VI.   References

7) Hahnemann, S. *Organon of Medicine, 6th Edition.*

8) *A dummies guide to LM potency.* (2008, october 16). Retrieved from Hpathy.com: http://hpathy.com/organon-philosophy/a-dummy%E2%80%99s-guide-to-lm-potencies/

9) B/K.Sarkar. (2011). *Hahnemann's Organon of Medicine.*

Homeopathic Approach and Therapeutics for Injuries

Chapter 4: Injuries to Soft Tissues

I.   Introduction

Soft tissue are the tissues that connect, support or surround other structures and the organs of the body. It includes ligaments, tendons, connective tissues, fibrous tissues and muscle. Soft tissue injuries are very common in people who are involved in sports and physical fitness activities.

Some of the soft tissue injuries are:[10]

- Bumps, bruises (contusions);
- small tear of muscles (minor strain);
- tear of ligaments and tendons (minor sprains).

These injuries occur due to fall, sudden twist of muscle, or blow to the body. Soft tissue injuries cause mild to moderate pain, swelling with discoloration of the injured part.[10]

II.   Bruises, Sprain and Strain

Contusion or bruise is usually caused due to a blow to the muscle, tendons or ligaments. The bruise is caused around the injury when the pool of blood sets or accumulates due to torn blood vessels. Due to accumulation of blood the injured part becomes purple or bluish in color. [10]

Most of the bruises are mild. Muscle contusion or bruise causes mild to moderate swelling and pain, with discoloration of the part and limit the range of motion near the injury.

Most of the contusions respond well to home treatment, however if the symptoms persists for longer time

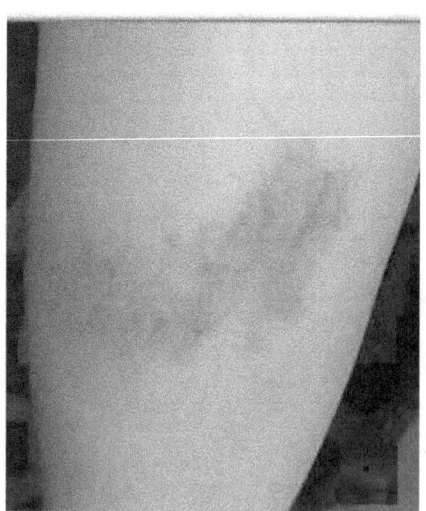

Bruise

Sprain and strains are common injuries that shows similar symptoms but involves different parts of the body. A Sprain is a tearing of ligaments, which is a band of connective tissue that joins the one end of bone with another. Most commonly sprain occurs in ankle, knee and wrist joint as these joint are more vulnerable than others. The sprain occurs mainly when you fall (sprain in wrist joint); and when you suddenly twist your ankle or knee (ankle or knee sprain). The twist of joint causes severe tension in the ligaments and may lead to mile to severe tear in the ligaments. The adjacent figure shows the mild, moderate and complete tear of ligament which can be compared with the normal ligament.

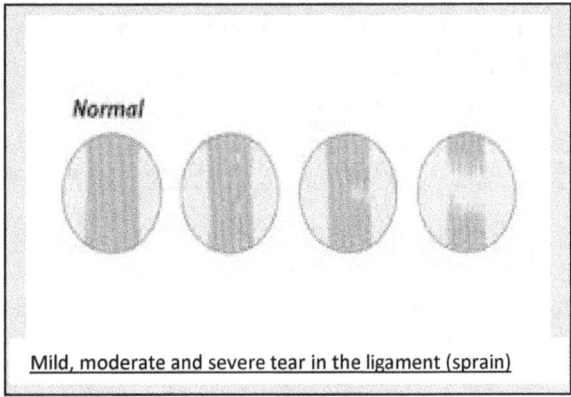
Normal

Mild, moderate and severe tear in the ligament (sprain)

Symptoms seen in sprain are pain, swelling, bruising if the sprain occurs due to fall, limited ability to move. At the time of injury you may hear a 'pop up' in your joint.[11]

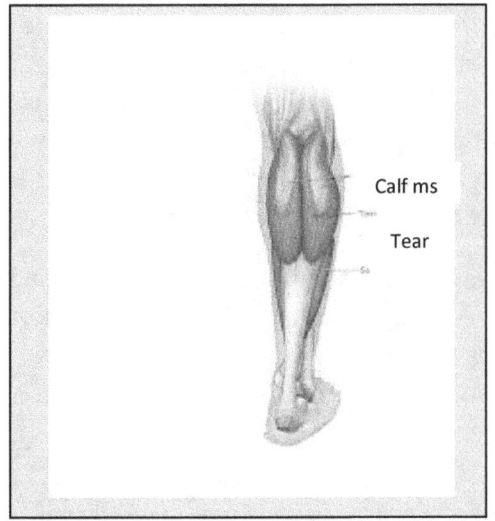
Calf ms

Tear

A Strain is an injury of a muscle and or tendon. Tendons are the fibrous tissues that attach muscles to bone. A strain results due to an injury to either a muscle or a tendon. Such injury may lead to either simple strain in the muscle or tendons, or it may be partial or complete tear in the muscle or tendons or both.[11]

Minor trauma to the tendons may cause only inflammation to it. However major injury like accidents can cause mild to moderate tear of tendons. The complete tear requires surgical repair.

Symptoms produced in case of strain are very similar to sprain, except there is no pop up feel in the joint, instead there will be muscle s

Muscle strain

III.   Treatment for soft tissue injuries

Mild sprains and contusions respond well to home treatment like compression, rest, cold application and elevation of the injured part. However if the injury is severe it needs medical help. Homeopathic treatment is very effective in treating injuries hence along with the general treatment, homeopathic approach would fasten the healing process and the recovery time.

i.   Common Homeopathic remedies for soft tissue injuries

Following are some of the commonly used homeopathic remedies, these remedies can be used along with the general modern medicine.

- **Arnica**

 The main theme of Arnica is deep trauma which can be either physical, mental or emotional trauma. Physical trauma can result from injuries, fall, or blow; mental or emotional trauma includes fright, fear, and financial loss. Arnica is frequently given in injuries especially due to blunt instruments which cause contusions and bruises with extravasation of blood from capillaries.

 Arnica is mainly indicated when patients complain of **sore and bruised feeling as if he has been beaten.** Due to soreness and pain, patient moves and appears restless. Arnica acts magically in soft tissue injuries after **over exertion of muscles**, for instance after heavy workout or exercise. I would administer Arnica if somebody gets blow and bruises on body due to fall from bike, or cycle. Even it works well after labor where women feels soreness after childbirth. Usually Arnica is not the remedy if tendons or muscles are sprained.

Dose: Arnica acts only if it is indicated and prescribed immediately after the injury. Arnica must be given orally within 24-48 hours of injuries. It can be given in 30C to 1M or higher repetitively or single dose depending on the acuteness of the complaints. For severe acute injuries, prescribe frequent doses of Arnica until the relief.

Following are some rubrics taken from Synthesis repertory 8.1 edition. These rubrics will help you understand the remedy in a better way.

Rubrics from Synthesis repertory 8.1 edition:

General- Injuries – blunt instruments from

General- Injuries – contusion

General- Injuries – extravasation with

General- Injuries – operation, ailments from

General – Injuries – deadness in bruised part; sensation of:

Female genitalia / sex - sore – labor after

- **Rhus Tox**

It is commonly indicated in sprains and strains due to over use of muscles and ligaments. Rhus Tox is very useful when tendons are inflamed either due to over exertion or from sudden wrenching. The patents mainly experiences **sprain and severe stiffness mainly in the morning which is better by hot bathing and continued motion.** Patient experiences aggravation from beginning of move however feels better with continued motion. Hence we find these patients more restless.

Rhus Tox acts magically by relieving the tension and spasm in the muscles or tendons. Rhus tox effectively heals the ruptured tendons (mild tear of muscle or tendons), however complete or severe tear of muscle or tendon may require surgical intervention and Rhus Tox may not be much useful.

Dose: 30 C and higher potency can be given orally with frequent repetition for acute injuries.

Rubrics from Synthesis repertory 8.1 edition:

Mind – morose – house agg; in / open air amel; on walking in

Mind – Restlessness – bed – driving out of

General – Injuries – Muscles, of

Generals – Injuries – rupture, tendons of

General – Injuries – sprains

General – wounds – swelling of

Extremities - Stiffness - moving-beginning to move on

Extremities - Stiffness - rising on

Extremities - Stiffness - walking after

Extremities - Stiffness – manual labor after

Extremities – Stiffness – exertion after

- **Bryonia**

Bryonia is another common indication for sprain and strain of muscles. Patients mainly complain of swelling, stiffness and pain in joints, which is aggravated by slightest motion (unlike Rhus Tox). Bryonia should be the first remedy to be thought of if pain and stiffness **ameliorates by lying down and suffers greatly on slightest motion.** The reason for this aggravation is excessive dryness of mucous membranes. Dryness in the mucous membranes produce less friction and restrict the free movements of joints, and muscles.

Dose: 30C to 1M can be given with some repetition. Do not repeat the dose frequently.

Rubrics from Synthesis repertory 8.1 edition:

Generals – Injuries – Overexertion, strain from

General – wounds – swelling of

Extremities- Sprains

Extremities – Swelling – joints

Extremities - Tension

- **Bellis Perennis**

Like Arnica, it is indicated in bruises and contusions, due to the external trauma where sore bruised feeling is marked with extravasation of blood, however less often indicated than Arnica. Bellis is mainly indicated when **the effects of fall or blow has turned into deep wound or septic wound**. If Arnica fails, Bellis Per is an effective remedy to manage the severe pain.

Dose: For acute conditions, administer 30C to 200C or higher potency, three to four times a day.

Rubrics from Synthesis repertory 8.1 edition:

General- Injuries – contusion

General- Injuries – Soft parts of

General- Injuries – extravasation with

General- Injuries – operation, ailments from

General- Injuries – sprain

General – wounds – lacerations

- **Ruta**

Ruta is another useful remedy for trauma and injury. It is indicated in **severe stiffness of muscles and tendons caused by trauma to the connective tissue or tendons**. It is a great remedy for ill-effects of carrying heavy load. When injury to periosteum, tendons, or muscle has occurred due to chronic over use of the part, Ruta is markedly indicated. Like Arnica, patient complains of sore bruised feeling in all the parts of the body due to stiffness in the muscles.

Dose: Ruta can be applied locally on closed wound to reduce the stiffness and pain. Ruta can be administered in 30C to 1M potency depending on the acuteness of the complaints.

Rubrics from Synthesis repertory 8.1 edition:

Generals – Injuries – Overexertion, strain from

Generals – Injuries - sprains

General – Injuries – Periosteum of

General – Injuries – Tendons of

Mind – Restlessness - feverish

IV.   Conclusion

- Soft tissue injury is commonly seen in everyday life. It includes injury to the muscles, tendons, ligaments and tissues (fibrous and connective tissues)

- Soft tissue injuries include bruises, sprains and strains which mainly caused by fall over the joint, sudden blow over the muscle, sudden twist of joint, etc. Pain, swelling, discoloration of the affected part, limited range of motion, muscle spasms are common signs and symptoms of soft tissue injuries.

- Although mild injuries respond well to the home treatment like rest, ice, compression, and elevation of the injured part, homeopathic approach effectively fastens the healing process. Hence with homeopathic approach the signs and symptoms does not last for longer time.

- Common homeopathic remedies indicated for soft tissue injuries are Arnica, Bellis Perrennis Rhus Toxicodedron and Ruta.

V.   References

10. *American Academy of Orthopaedic Surgeons*. (2007). Retrieved from Orthoinfo: http://orthoinfo.aaos.org/topic.cfm?topic=A00304

11. Corp, M. S. (2009-2015). *Merck Manual Hom Edition*. Retrieved from Merck Manuals: http://www.merckmanuals.com/home/injuries_and_poisoning/first_aid/soft-tissue_injuries.html

Chapter 5: Nerve Injury

I.   Introduction

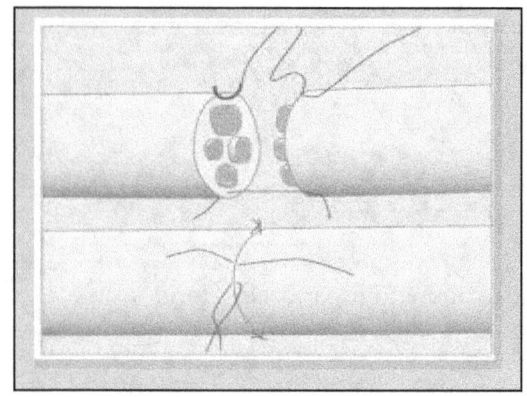

Nerve Injury

'Nerves' acts like a wire of the body that carry information to and from the brain. Nerves are sensitive and fragile, can be damaged by pressure, cutting or stretching. Any injury to a nerve can stop signals to and from brain, causing dysfunction of muscles. [12]

II.   Types of Nerves

There are three types of nerves that carry message to the muscles and different body parts.[12] (MD, 2005-2015)

- Autonomic nerves control the involuntary or partially voluntary activities of the body, including heart rate, digestion, blood pressure and temperature regulation. For instance, diabetic autonomic neuropathy affects the digestive system.
- Motor nerves carry message between brain and spinal cord to the muscles.
- Sensory nerves carry signal from muscles back to brain and that information is processed to let you feel the sensations, pain or pressure.

Pressure on the nerves can cause the nerve fiber to break, may interfere with the ability to send or receive the message to and from the brain. If the nerve is severely damaged and not fixed, the growing nerve fibers may produce severe pain called as 'neuroma'.

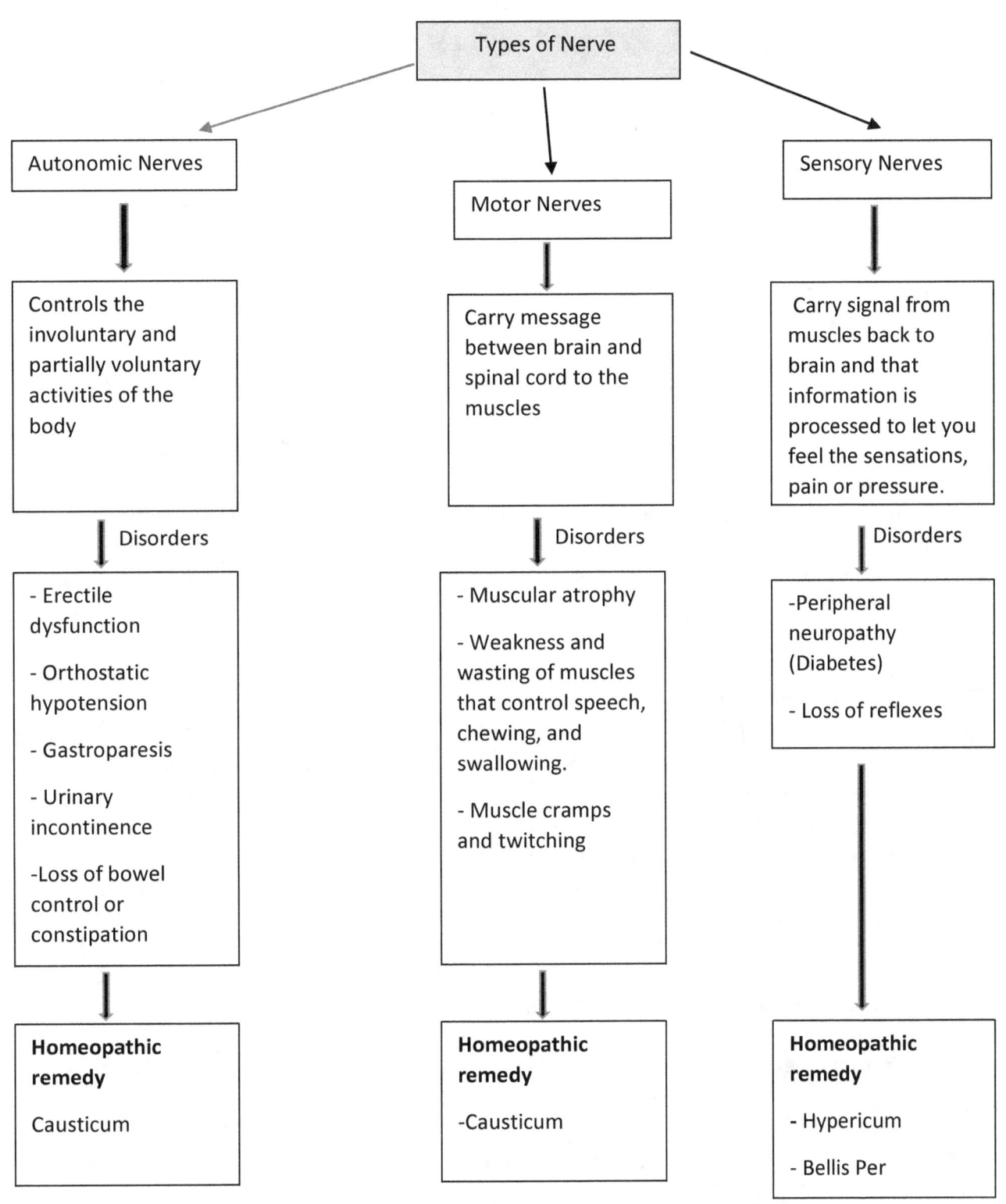

Types of Nerve

Autonomic Nerves

Controls the involuntary and partially voluntary activities of the body

Disorders

- Erectile dysfunction

- Orthostatic hypotension

- Gastroparesis

- Urinary incontinence

-Loss of bowel control or constipation

Homeopathic remedy

Causticum

Motor Nerves

Carry message between brain and spinal cord to the muscles

Disorders

- Muscular atrophy

- Weakness and wasting of muscles that control speech, chewing, and swallowing.

- Muscle cramps and twitching

Homeopathic remedy

-Causticum

Sensory Nerves

Carry signal from muscles back to brain and that information is processed to let you feel the sensations, pain or pressure.

Disorders

-Peripheral neuropathy (Diabetes)

- Loss of reflexes

Homeopathic remedy

- Hypericum

- Bellis Per

There are several possible causes for nerve injury or nerve damage. They are listed below –

1. Direct injury to the nerves due to compression or trauma.
2. Diabetes – Diabetic neuropathy is serious complication of diabetes. It affects all the three types of nerves. However sensory nerves are most commonly affected.
3. Autoimmune diseases: Diseases like multiple sclerosis, and Guillain-Barré syndrome, etc can damage the nerves causing nerve pain.
4. Cancer: Cancerous mass can push or compress the nerve and can cause nerve damage.
5. Motor Neuron diseases: Certain diseases including Amyotrophic Lateral Sclerosis (AML) can damage the motor neurons
6. Nutritional Deficiencies: Deficiency of certain vitamins like Vitamin B6 and B12 can produce the symptoms of nerve pain, with burning and tingling sensation.

III.   Treatment for nerve injuries

Treatment depends on the cause of the nerve injury. If the nerve is severely damaged due to cut, nerve regeneration is strongly recommended. This becomes an emergency and need immediate attention. Along with emergency treatment, homeopathic remedy can act wonderfully to speed the recovery of the wound healing. Remember following remedies will only help to curb the acute condition of the patient. However for complete cure, deeper understanding of the cause of disease and similimum remedy is required.

i.   Homeopathic management for nerve injuries

- **Hypericum**
  It is a great remedy for injuries to the nerves especially of fingers, toes and nails; and spine. Hypericum has special affinity towards puncture wounds, lacerations and crushing injuries with severe nerve damage. **The hallmark of Hypericum is sharp, shooting type of pain**. It makes a great remedy even for injuries to brain and spinal cord. This remedy works well for sensory nerve disorders like peripheral nerve damage due to diabetes. It relieves the sharp pain after surgeries and post anesthesia.

  Dose: In acute painful stage, you can prescribe Hypericum 30c to 1M every 15 to 30 minutes then gradually reduce the frequency of repetition to once a day.

  Rubrics from Synthesis Repertory 8.1:

  Extremities - Injuries – nerves - sentient

  Extremities – Injuries - nerves - fracture with laceration

  General - Injuries – nerves of – pain with great

- **Bellis Per**
Bellis is mainly indicated when the effects of fall or blow has turned into deep wound or septic wound affecting the nerves. It works well when result on injuries to nerves with intense soreness and intolerance of cold bathing.

Dose: Bellis Per 200C or higher can be prescribed two to three times a day or more frequently if the condition is acute.

- **Causticum**
Causticum works effectively for **motor neuron diseases** where injury to motor nerve leads to muscular atrophy, emaciation of extremities and paralysis. Commonly indicated in paralysis of flexor muscles after cerebral accidents and neuro-degenerative disorders. Strongly indicated in right sided facial paralysis, and Bell's Palsy, aggravated from draft of cold air or winds.
Causticum has been effective in treating autonomic nerve disorders like urinary incontinence, erectile dysfunction, etc.
Along with the physical complaints, Causticum patients will show strong history of repeated grief and depressions. Most of the complaints aggravate or arise in situations of intense or suppressed emotions.

Dose: Causticum should be prescribed in 30C to 1M potency with less frequent repetition.

Rubrics from Synthesis Repertory 8.1:
Generals – Emaciation – Single parts of
Generals – Paralysis – Muscles - Flexor muscles of
Generals – Paralysis – Organs of – Single pars of
Generals – Paralysis Agitans
Generals – Paralysis – air / draft of air or wind, after

IV. Conclusion

- Nerves are essential part of the body. Injury to nerve in any form can be serious with lifelong complications.

- Autonomic nerve control the involuntary or partially voluntary activities of the body, including heart rate, digestion, blood pressure and temperature regulation. Damage of autonomic nerve cause erectile dysfunction, urine incontinence, loss of bowel movements, orthostatic hypotension, etc.

- Motor Nerve carry message between brain and spinal cord to the muscles. Damage to motor nerve leads to muscular atrophy, weakness and numbness of muscles, muscle cramps and tingling.

- Sensory nerve carry signal from muscles back to brain and that information is processed to let you feel the sensations, pain or pressure. Damage of sensory nerve leads to neurological disorders like diabetic neuropathy, peripheral neuropathy, loss of reflexes.

- If the nerve is severely damaged as a completed or partial cut (seen in accidental injuries) then surgical nerve regeneration is the only option. However further management after the surgery can be effectively treated with Homeopathic approach.

- Common homeopathic remedies for nerve injuries are Hypericum, Bellis Per, and Causticum.

V.   References

12. MD, W. (2005-2015). *Nerve pain and nerve damage*. Retrieved from Web MD: http://www.webmd.com/brain/nerve-pain-and-nerve-damage-symptoms-and-causes.

Chapter 6: Bone Injury / Dislocations and Fractures

I. Introduction

Dislocation and Fracture are two common bone injuries. Dislocation and fracture are two different terms with different meanings. Dislocation is the separation or displacement of joints. It means two bones are out of place at joint that connects them. Dislocation may cause injury to nerves and blood vessels. Fracture is a break or crack in the bone. Any severe injury to bone can lead to compound fracture or open fracture. The bone fragments of this fractured bone may penetrate the surface of the skin and may produce wound infection if persists for longer time. Never try to straighten the bone at this time as this can increase the possibility of infection due to dirt and other surrounding particles.

II. Causes, Signs and symptoms

Fractures are caused when too much pressure is put on the bone which breaks the bone. Common cause of fracture includes fall, accident, blow, or any mechanical injuries. Stress fracture are common too, where repetitive pressure is put on the particular bone. Deficiency of vitamin D and Calcium can lead to fracture as bone becomes so brittle that they break even without any pressure.

Fracture or dislocation can lead to tenderness, swelling, and discoloration at the site of injury. Also deformity of injured part is common. Patient may lose sensation due to injury to the nerves.

III. Treatment for bone injuries

Immediate medical attention is required in case of dislocation or fracture. First apply the ice pack at the site of fracture and dislocation. It will reduce the swelling and stop the blood flow in case if blood vessel is cut.

Then do not try to align the fracture bone as it may cause more damage. Instead splint the injured part so that it doesn't move.

Transfer the patient to nearby hospital for further management.

i. Homeopathic management for bone injuries:

Homeopathically we can manage the patient by speeding the recovery of the fractured bones and help to relieve the pain. Certain remedies work very effectively in bone injuries. They are:

- **Symphytum**

  Symphytum is an excellent remedy for fractures and mechanical injuries on the bones with excessive pain. It accelerates the reunion of bone, lessens the pain and favors the production of callous. It is also useful in cases of painful old injuries where pain remains after wound has healed. However remember, Symphytum does not act all the time. It will act only when the symptoms calls for.

  Dose: In case of fracture, I always prescribe Arnica 30 C or 200 C for immediate relief from soreness after trauma for couple of days depending on the patient's discomfort, followed by Symphytum 30C or 200C on repetitive basis till the bone heals.

  Rubrics from Synthesis Repertory 8.1 edition:

  - Generals – Injuries – dislocation
  - Generals – Injuries – Periosteum of
  - General - Injuries – Bones – fractures of
  - Generals – Brittle bones
  - General - Injuries – Bones – fractures of; slow repair of broken bones

- **Ruta graveolens**

  Ruta is another useful remedy when injury has occurred to periosteum, connective tissues and tendons. It is a great remedy for ill-effects of carrying heavy load. When injury to periosteum has occurred due to chronic over use of the part, Ruta is markedly indicated. Ruta is indicated when patient complains of injury with severe stiffness in the muscles and tendons. Like Arnica, patient complains of sore bruised feeling in all the parts of the body. In case of dislocation or fracture when the inflammation is under control, it hastens the curative process in the joint. Dose: Ruta can be applied locally on closed wound to reduce the stiffness and pain. I would administer this remedy in low to higher potency.

  Rubrics from Synthesis Repertory 8.1 edition:

  General - Injuries – Bones – fractures of; slow repair of broken bones

  General - Injuries – Bones – fractures of; Compound fracture

  General – Injuries – Periosteum of

  General – Injuries – Tendons of

- **Silicea**

  Silicea is nearly indicated in the diseases of bone. It is a great remedy for healing the fracture as it efficiently metabolizes the calcium and vitamin D towards the healing of injured bone.

  If the fragments of bone are penetrated deep into the wound and very difficult to remove them, Silicea will work towards it. It ripens abscess and promotes suppuration.

  Dose: To promote the suppuration in bone injuries, prescribe Silicea 200 or 1M three times a day. Silicea can be prescribed in lower potency of 6X or 12X twice a day until the fractured bone heals.

  Rubrics from Synthesis Repertory 8.1 edition:

  Generals – Brittle bones

  Extremities – Abscess – Bones – Joints

IV. Conclusion

- Injury to bone is very commonly seen in children as their bones are not very strong hence they are more vulnerable for dislocations and fractures.

- Dislocation and fracture are two common bone injuries. Dislocation is the separation or displacement of joints. Fracture is a break or crack in the bone.

- Fracture or dislocation can lead to tenderness, swelling, and discoloration at the site of injury. Also deformity of injured part is common. Patient may lose sensation due to injury to the nerves.

- Cold application at the site of fracture or dislocation helps to reduce the swelling and pain.

- In case of fracture never try to straighten the bone as this can increase the possibility of infection due to dirt and other surrounding particles.

- Along with surgical and medical attention, Homeopathic approach effectively fastens the recovery period.

- Common homeopathic remedies for bone injuries are Arnica, Calcarea Flouricum, Symphytum, Ruta and Silicea

Chapter 7: Bees, Insects and Animal Bites

I.   Introduction

Insect bites and bee stings cause mild to severe allergic reactions. Bites from bees, mosquitoes, ticks, flies, scorpion, spiders, dogs, and snakes are troublesome, and cause allergic reactions. The allergic reactions are due to the release of venomous substance into the skin after the bites. The severity of the reaction depends on the individual sensitivity to the venom.

II.   Signs and Symptoms

Most of the insect bites like mosquitoes, ticks produce mild reactions (immediate) like itching or stinging sensation with mild swelling at the site of bite or sting. This reaction last for a day or so and then it disappears.

Some individuals suffer from delayed reaction like fever, hives, swollen glands and painful joints. Small percentage of people suffer from severe reactions like facial swelling, swelling all over body, difficulty in breathing and loss of consciousness.

Dog bite is very common too. Children are more likely to be injured by a dog bite. Dog bite can cause punctured, and a lacerated wound at the site of injury. If the infected dog bites it can lead to sepsis, infection to brain and other internal organs. Severe pain, redness and swelling around the bite. High grade fever and abscess or pus at the site of bite. If the skin is broken from a dog bite it can allow the bacteria that causes tetanus, *Clostridium tetani,* to enter the skin. Symptoms appear after four to 21 days and include muscle stiffness and spasms.[13]

III.   Treatment for bees sting, insect and animal bites

Mild reaction to bee sting or animal bites (except snake bite or scorpion bite are highly venomous) don't need special treatment as the reaction goes away in few hours. Follow few steps at home to relieve the pain and temporary allergic reaction.

- Wash and clean the area where the bees or insect bit you.
- It is important to remove the stinger stuck into the skin in order prevent the further release of venom or toxic substance.
- Apply ice pack to the painful area.

- Encourage bleeding from the bleeding site, if it is not bleeding then gently squeeze the wound to encourage it to bleed, which will help prevent bacteria entering the wound.

Recurrent severe reaction requires the treatment because recurrent allergic reaction may affect the immune system and may not respond to the home treatment very well. Severe allergic reaction can be fatal. Hence immediate attention is required if the symptoms remain for linger time or get worsen in 5-6 hours of insect bit.

Infected dog bite and snake bite requires immediate medical treatment before the infection and venom spreads to all the internal organs. Here in short I will be discussing the management for snake bite as small bite can take away the breath in short span of time.

Management for snake bite:

- Apply tight band (rubber band, or piece of cloth), 2-3 inches above the bitten spot to restrict the superficial venous blood flow. Loosen the band every 15 min for 60-75 seconds & tie it again just above the spreading area
- Apply ice or cold pack on and around the wound.
- Remove the snake venom from the bitten site by using suction; suction can be done in two ways. Firstly, if a suction pump is available then this method can be useful. Make a sterile incision, of approximately 1 cm long & 0.5 cm deep. Clean the wound with water or weak potassium permanganate. Use suction pump to remove the venom from the wound.
  If suction pump is not available, second method can be used. In this case, suction can be done by mouth. Make sure there are no open ulcers or oral wound.
- Continue suction for 15 minutes every one hour until toxic fluid stops coming out.
- Cover the wound with sterile cloth
- Next aim is to neutralize the venom by injecting antivenin. To achieve maximum efficacy, administer it within 4-6 hours of the bite.
- Homeopathic approach for snake bite poisoning can be very helpful as homeopathic remedy not only effective in neutralizing the toxicity of venom but will also prevent the complications associated with the snake bite.
- However in snake bite cases, first aid treatment should be the priority and later homeopathically it can be treated. Based on the symptoms homeopathic remedies can be given. Some commonly indicated remedies are described below.

i.   Homeopathic remedies for bees sting, insect and animal bites
- **Apis Mellifica**
  Apis Mellifica is very well known to revert the anaphylactic shock after bee sting. Apis is indicated when an individual suffers from **burning, stinging pain, redness, hives and swelling, after bee sting and insect bite.**
  It works well in case of localized and generalized edema (anasarca) and urticaria due to allergic reaction. Often, it **is better by cold application and intolerant to heat and slightest touch.** Also, such individual will complain of sensation of stiffness and as of something torn off in the interior of the body. Generally this individual is **thirstless during the complaints.**

Dose: 30C to 1M or higher potency with repetition should be useful in acute conditions. Single dose or less frequent repetition in chronic conditions.

Rubrics from Synthesis Repertory 8.1 edition:

Generals – Dropsy – general in – eruption, from suppressed

Generals – Dropsy – general in – overexertion agg

Generals – Dropsy – general in – thirst, without

Generals – Dropsy – internal drops – serous membranes

Generals – wounds – penetrating, punctured

- **Ledum Palustra**
  Ledum is a well-known acute remedy in bites, stings and wounds. Immediately administer Ledum in bites from insects like spiders, mosquitoes; animal bites like dog and snake; and stings. Remember to administer Ledum in penetrating, punctured wounds like injury due a dog bite, where bleeding is very less but with severe pain and the affected part becomes cold.
  Here hypericum can be compared with Ledum as both have very similar symptomatology.
  Ledum and Hypericum both helps to prevent tetanus after the injuries. The most striking feature of Ledum pal is the amelioration of the complaints by cold application, swollen, red purple and mottled part; and punctured, stabbing wound.
  Ledum works well when Arnica fails to clear the bruises and ecchymosis.

Dose: In case of serious animal bites, administer high repetitive dose of the remedy. Ledum Pal 200C and higher can be given 3-4 times a day until the symptoms reduces in intensity.

Rubrics from Synthesis Repertory 8.1 edition

Generals – Injury – tetanus; prophylaxis of

Generals – Wounds – bites

Generals – Wounds – bites - poisonous animals, of

Generals – Wounds – bites – snakes

Generals – Wounds – cold, become

Generals – Wounds – injection; from painful

Generals – Wounds – penetrating, punctured

Generals – Injury – tetanus prophylaxis of

- **Lachesis**

  Lachesis is well known for treating animal bites especially snake bites. If the wound changes its color to purple with full plethoric appearance, Lachesis is the remedy. The discoloration is due to lack of blood supply to the part, Lachesis will restore the blood supply to some extent. Lachesis will also antidote the effect if snake bite. Before prescribing any remedy make sure to go for first aid treatment for snake bite which includes placing the constrictive band 2-3 inches above and below the bite and do not elevate the part.

  Dose: Lachesis 30C orally at frequent interval will help to reduce the discoloration, pain and bleeding. Ledum Pal 1M and Hypericum 1M can be prescribed alternatively with Lachesis 30C if the symptoms matches.

  Rubrics from Synthesis Repertory 8.1 edition:
  Generals – Wounds – snakes of
  Generals – Wounds – bluish
  Generals – Wounds – cuts
  Generals – Wounds – gangrene of
  Generals – Wounds – heal tendency to, slowly

IV. Conclusion

- Dog bite is very commonly seen. Children are more likely to be injured by a dog bite. If a dog is not infected, the home treatment is sufficient to recover from the injury. However if a dog is infected immediate medical attention is necessary.

- Snake bite is always dangerous and also very difficult to save the life of the individual unless immediate action is taken. Homeopathic remedy may not act very quickly and hence such patients require quick medical treatment. Some homeopathic remedy like Lachesis may act as anti-venom.

- Insect bite and bee stings produce immediate mild to moderate local allergic reaction. Some individuals suffer from delayed reaction like fever, hives, swollen glands and painful joints. And small number of people suffer from severe reactions like facial swelling, swelling all over body, difficulty in breathing and loss of consciousness.

- First aid treatment is must in animal and insect bites. First aid helps to reduce the further exposure to infection or toxins.

- Some homeopathic remedies like Apis, Lachesis, Ledum Pal, Urtica Ureans, Tarentula, etc can be helpful. Prescribe the remedies based in the symptoms and cause of the injury.

V.   References

13. *Dog Bites*. Retrieved from Web MD: http://pets.webmd.com/dogs/dog-bites.

Chapter 8: Burns and Blisters

I.   Introduction

Burn is a common household injury caused by exposure to heat or flame which causes severe skin damage or death of affected cells. Most of the time household burns are minor and home treatment is able to restore the damaged skin cells. Most of the time women are the victim of kitchen burns. Such burns can be treated at home very easily. However the most serious burn require immediate medical attention in order to prevent further infection.

II.   Classification and Degree of Burn

Let us first understand how the burns are classified. Following chart gives the brief overview of the types of burn.[14]

Classification and degree of Burn		
First Degree	**Second degree**	**Third Degree**
• Red, non blistered skin • Superficial burn • Pain • Usually heals in 3-6 days	• Blisters and thickening of skin • Wet appearance burn • Damage extends beyoud the superficial layer of skin	• Widespread thickness with leathery appearance of skin • Serious deep burn • Less painful burn
Homeopathic remedy • Urtica Ureans • Calendula	Homeopathic remedy • Hypericum • Calendula	Homeopathic remedy • Cantharis • Arsenic Album

There are several causes of burns. Some of them are:[14]

- Scalding burns from hot liquid are the most common burns to children and older adults
- Fire flames due to candles, lighters, etc
- Electricity burns are caused by contact with electricity or lightening
- Chemical burns are caused by contact with household or industrial chemicals like misuse of hair or skin products; or use of strong acids or strong bases.
- Radiation burn is caused by excessive exposure to sun, tanning, x-rays or radiation therapy for cancer, etc.

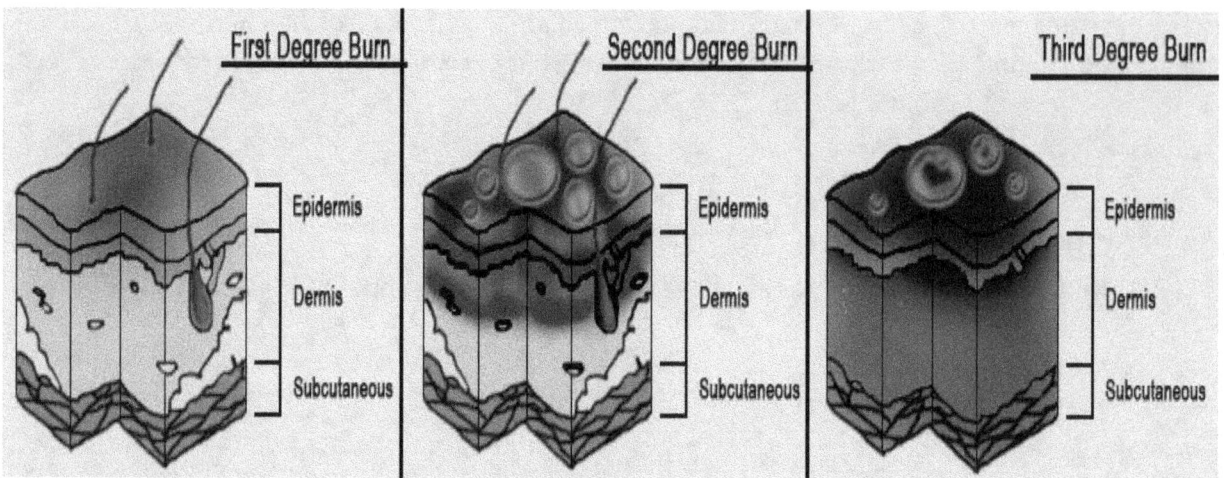

Degree of Burn

III.   Common homeopathic treatment for burn

Whether its minor or deep burn, it needs immediate attention. Fortunately, most of the minor or superficial burns are treatable at home. Homeopathic treatment helps to alleviate the pain, regenerate the new skin cells and hastens the recovery time. Homeopathic remedies are prescribed based on the level of injuries. For first and second degree burn apply the calendula and Urtica Ureans cream and apply loose bandage. Remember do not apply tight bandage in case of burn as tightness may increase the risk of infection.

- **Urtica Ureans**
  This remedy has been used primarily for its beneficial effects on skin, and for conditions like urticaria, allergic reaction due to bee stings, and burns. Urtica Ureans can be used as a remedy in **first degree burns**. Swelling and blisters occur after the burn with severe stinging pain. It relieves the pain of first degree burn, even sun burn. Hence it is primary remedy for sun burn.

  Dose: Urtica Ureans can be applied locally in the form of diluted tincture or ointment at the affected part. It can be taken internally in 6c, 30c or 200c potency.

Rubrics from Synthesis Repertory 8.1 edition:

Skin – Eruptions – Urticaria

Skin – Eruptions – Urticaria – alternating with rheumatism

Skin – Eruptions – blisters – burn; as from a

Skin – Eruptions – sun; from

- **Calendula:**

 I call Calendula as a multipurpose homeopathic remedy and of the best remedy for open wound injuries. It is known as **homeopathic antiseptic** because it rapidly heals the tissue before infection sets in. This remedy is useful in **first and second degree burns** where blisters and vesicles have developed around the burnt area. Calendula soothes the burnt part and promote regeneration of skin cells.

Calendula is indicated mainly in lacerated, incised and sometimes in punctured wound where the skin is torn. Remember, when skin is not torn, and external trauma only produces extravasation of blood, Arnica acts magically. However when the skin is torn and inflammation sets it, Calendula is the best remedy.

Dose: Local applications in minor injuries or burn. I have personally used calendula cream for first degree burn. You can use it for dressing the wound too, it acts magically.

If the infection has already set in the wound or at the site of burn, internal dose of 200c or 1M promotes fast healing.

You can also directly apply the diluted tincture of calendula (10 drops of tincture in a cup of water) three times a day.

Rubrics from Synthesis Repertory 8.1 edition:

Generals – Wounds – bleeding freely

Generals – Wounds – cuts

Generals – Wounds – foreign bodies from

Generals – Wounds –lacerations

Generals – Wounds – soft tissues; with torn

Generals – Wounds - suppurating

- **Cantharis**

  This remedy is mainly indicated in **second or third degree burn** and scald burn where severe burning pain has set in with severe inflammation and over sensitiveness of the part. Burning is so severe that patient gets restless and goes into delirium.

  Patient is usually better by application of cold water, however excess and sudden application of cold water may worsen the burns. It relieves the severe burning pain following a burn, and helps to promote the healing of the wound. Cantharis works well in severe sun burns too.

  Dose: For second and third degree burn, immediate medical attention is necessary. Along with calendula, apply cantharis externally. It can be taken internally in 30C potency.

  Rubrics from Synthesis Repertory 8.1 edition:

  Generals – Inflammation – gangrenous – tendency to

  Skin – Eruptions – blisters

  Skin – Eruptions – blisters – burn as from a

- **Causticum**

  It is indicated in the burns which takes long time to heal. If the burnt part has not healed properly, or old wound starts to reopen or gets re-infected, Causticum is the remedy. Causticum mainly works in **second degree burn**.

  Remember causticum is rarely indicated as primary burn remedy. Causticum will work if it is a similimum remedy.

  Dose: Depending on the patient's susceptibility and case history, Causticum can be indicated in 30C to 1M potency.

  Rubrics from Synthesis Repertory 8.1 edition:

  General – Burns – heals slowly.

  General – wounds – reopening of old – cicatrices

- **X-Ray**

  I have never used this remedy till now. However seen some homeopaths using it successfully. X-ray is a remedy indicated in burns caused due to repetitive exposure to radiation of x-rays. This remedy works well when skin lesions are deep, obstinate, and wounds are difficult to heal. X-ray is a constitutional remedy and will act only if the symptomatology matches.

  Dose: Single dose of 30C or higher potency can be prescribed. Some homeopaths prescribe frequent repetitions of this remedy in lower potencies.

Rubrics from Synthesis Repertory 8.1 edition:

Generals – Burns – x-ray from

IV. Conclusion

- First degree burn is 'superficial burn' as it damages the superficial or the top layer of the skin. It is characterized by redness, pain, and mild swelling with no blisters.

- Second degree burn is serious kind of burn as it damages the beyond the top or superficial layer of the skin. This kind of extensive damage causes blister over the skin.

- Third degree burn is the serious kind of deep burn because damage extends through all layers of the skin to the internal organs, blood vessels, and bones. It may even cause death.

- For minor burn, hold the burnt part in lukewarm running water (not cold water as it will cause more damage). If the blisters break wash the part with water and apply ointment like calendula and cover it with non-stick gauge bandage.

- Homeopathic approach is very effective to treat the minor burns. Common homeopathic remedies for burns are Calendula, Hypericum, Urtica ureans, Cantharis, Caustisum, X-rays. Remedies like Calendula, Hypericum and Urtica ureans can be taken orally and applied locally as well.

V. References

14. Plus, M. (2015, 2 12). *Burns*. Retrieved from US National Library of Medicine and National Institute of Health: http://www.nlm.nih.gov/medlineplus/ency/article/000030.htm.

Chapter 9: Surgical Wounds

I. Introduction

In conventional medicine, surgery represents one of the greatest achievement in medicine. With the advent of technology in the field of medicine, surgery has become an easier effort to remove the disease and prevent further disease complications. However the surgeries has its own pros and cons. An advanced technology has helped surgeons to perform the surgeries with minimal invasion. Surgical intervention in emergency and life threatening conditions can save a life of many. Intervention of both surgery and Homeopathy together hand in hand would make success in treating the patients. For instance, in case of injury from severe accidents, lightening, congenital deformities, etc will need immediate attention to arouse the vitality of an individual. Here Homeopathy will not work due to lack of vitality in the patients. Homeopathic remedy will act once the vitality is significantly aroused. Hence homeopathy will work magically after intervention.

Surgical intervention is very important to remove the mechanical cause or external factors. For instance, if a person has injured his eyes due to foreign body, the first step is to remove that foreign body through the surgery. In this case homeopathic medicine will not work unless the external factor is removed. Homeopathic remedy can work very well in the process of healing.

II. Surgical wounds

Usually surgery acts as only palliative mode of treatment because it suppresses the disease by acting against the vital force. Even though technology is advanced today, it cannot reduce the malady of the patients before and after the surgeries. For many people going through a surgery is a major process. The people has to go through pre and post-operative trauma which is completely unavoidable. For instance laproscopic cholecystectomy (laproscopic removal of gall bladder). This surgery is performed in a less invasive way to remove gall bladder. Many surgeons are highly skilled in performing these kind of surgeries. However many patients go through various kind of troubles like anxiety before surgery and delayed wound healing, secondary infection, bleeding, bruises, etc. These pre and post effects of surgeries are preventable by homeopathy. I don't want to criticize any surgical interventions as in some cases surgery is essential and the only option as there is limited scope of homeopathy in the field of surgery. For instance, Hernias are not treatable by homeopathy (however it is preventable), in such cases surgery is the only option to treat the patient. However a homeopathic remedy would help to prevent the post-surgical trauma and further occurrences of the same disease.

Homeopathic remedies before and after surgical interventions would definitely help to alleviate fear and anxiety before the surgery; and pain, bruising, bleeding, etc after the surgery. These remedies would prevent further complications, and scaring associated with the surgery. Most of the time people complain of bloating and nausea after surgery, it is due to the effect of anesthesia, can be managed by homeopathy as well.

III.   Treatment for surgical wounds

Here are some common homeopathic remedies that can be useful in the pre-operative and post-operative surgical wounds.

i.   Pre-operative injuries

Modern medicine usually prescribe anti-anxiety medication prior to the surgery so that patient sleep well at night remains calm next day for the surgery. However such medications don't work all the time. Homeopathic medicines have been useful is treating pre-operative anxieties and fear. Pre-operative injuries are not the external injuries, but it's mainly the mental injury which is represented in the form of fear and anxiety of going through the scary process. I have seen many patients in the hospitals having panic attacks one night before the surgery. Some of them suffer from physical ailments prior to surgery like low grade fever, diarrhea, trembling, etc. These physical ailments are due to anxiety and fear of surgical process. In such case I would advise to take the mental and physical picture of the individual and prescribe accordingly. Individualization and selection of correct similimum are the important aspect of treating homeopathicwise.

Some common remedies for pre-operative injuries are as follows:

- **Aconite**
  Aconite is commonly indicated when a person has intense fear and anxiety of going through surgery. Most of the time such people would say that they will die during the surgery. This kind of reaction is commonly seen in young children and elderly people. **Fear of death with severe anxiety is common indication of Aconite**. Administer Aconite 30C single dose at night before the surgery. Repeat the dose if patient complains of the same fear and anxiety.

- **Gelsemium**
  This is a very common remedy and very close to Aconite. It is indicated when a person has **great anxiety with weakness feeling, trembling of body and apprehension before surgery**. Such patient are usually dull and drowsy. Gelsemium 30C can be given a night before the surgery.

- **Arnica**
  Arnica can be taken just prior to the minor or major surgeries. For instance, Arnica 200C can be taken 2-3 hours before dental surgeries. Pre-operative administration of Arnica effectively

reduces and limits the inflammation and bleeding during surgery. It will also give instant relief from pain.

ii.   Post-operative injuries

Post-operative injuries are very common even though the surgery is done very well. Usually surgeons and physicians start with antibiotics immediately after the surgery to prevent and treat the post-operative infection.

Common post-operative injury includes excessive bleeding especially after prostrate surgery or root canal; scarring due to incision, pain at the site of spinal anesthesia, bruises due to cut for incision into deep and superficial muscles; and secondary post-operative infection of wound. Homeopathic remedies act very well in post-operative wounds too. But remember the remedy and potency should be prescribed based on the intensity of symptoms and patient's condition. Do not continue these medicine for longer time (more than 2 days).

Some common remedies that Homeopath can effectively use post-operatively are as follows:

- **Arnica**
  Arnica acts well in post-operative wounds too. Arnica 30C or 200C or even higher can be given after surgery to stop the bleeding. Arnica should be given when there is bruising and soreness of the tissue with swelling after the surgery. Some homeopaths use Arnica as prophylactic for pus infection. The potency and frequency of repetition of Arnica depends on the intensity of pain, and intensity of symptoms.

  Rubrics from Synthesis Repertory 8.1 edition:

  Generals – Wounds – suppurating, prophylaxis of pus infection.

- **Bellis Per**
  This remedy is very effective when **bruising and injury occurs to the deep tissue or muscles after surgery of breast or abdomen. It is indicated mainly in trauma which is followed by coldness of the part.** Bellis per is useful to alleviate the pain after surgery and to speed the healing process. It should be given in 30C potency, two or three times a day till the pain reduces.

- **Hypericum**
  Hypericum is very effective **after spinal anesthesia** where patient experience severe sharp shooting pain at the site of anesthesia. It is useful to relieve the pain after spinal surgery where lot of nerves are involved. Hypericum should be given in 30C or in higher potency, thrice a day or frequently for 1-2 days. Hypericum can be applied externally to prevent the wound infection.

- **Staphysagria**

  It is one of the remedy for incised wound where wounds are sharp cut-like and caused by knife or bullet. It should be taken in 30C or 200C potency, every 4-5 hourly until the symptom lessens.

- **Calendula**

  Calendula works effectively in the bed sores and infection at the sutured site. It acts very well both internally and as well as externally. Externally it can be applied over the sutured area to prevent infection. If the infection sets in, wound dressing can be done with calendula ointment. It will reduce the infection immediately. Dressing should be done 2-3 times every day. Oral administration of Calendula 30C or 200Calong with external application promotes quick healing of wounds.

- **Hamamelis**

  It is an effective remedy when the patient has varicose veins or hemorrhoids with sore, bruised sensation. Easy bleeding of veins due to weakness is an indication of this remedy. Hamamelis mainly effective to reduce the excessive venous bleeding. It can be taken orally internally in 30C potency, twice a day.

- **Hepar Sulphuricum**

  Hepar Sulphuricum is a best choice in post-surgical infection especially after the surgery of abdomen or spine. Hepar Sulphuricum is usually indicated when abscess develops into the wound after surgery. It helps to reduce the infection and pus. But remember do not administer in freshly sutured wounds because Hepar sulphuricum has an ability to expulse the foreign body. Here surgical stitches can act as foreign object, it may expulse the stitches. Hence administer it in open wound. If the wound has abscess in it, give Hepar sulp in 30C or 200C potency.

  Such patients are exquisitely sensitive to pain and are vulnerable to recurrent infections. Infection comes easily in the form of pus, sepsis, and fever.

- **Nux Vomica**

  Whenever a person complains of violent eructation's, and nauseous feeling but no vomiting after few hours of surgery, prescribe Nux Vomica 30 C or 200 C every 4 hourly till the symptoms reduces.

  Here are some general rubrics in reference to this remedy:

  Rubrics from Synthesis Repertory 8.1 edition:

  Stomach – Nausea – dinner after

  Stomach – Nausea – eating after

  Stomach – Nausea – inability to vomit

Stomach – vomiting – food

- **Ipecac**

  If a person vomits with severe nauseous feeling and headache, without relief after vomiting, Ipecac is an indicated remedy. Administer Ipecac 30 C, every 4 hourly till the symptoms subsides.

  Rubrics from Synthesis Repertory 8.1 edition:

  Stomach – vomiting – constant

  Stomach – vomiting – food

- **Carbo vegatabilis**

  This remedy is indicative if the post-surgery patient complains of bloating and gas feeling in the stomach and constantly produce eructation's, however ameliorates after eructations. Such patient will also ask for fresh air or fanning after surgery even though the surrounding is cold. Carbo veg 30C or 200C can be taken orally thrice a day.

  Rubrics from Synthesis Repertory 8.1 edition:

  Abdomen – distension – eructations amel

  Abdomen – distension – flatus, passing amel

- **Pyrogen**

  Pyrogen is well-known for treating the acute conditions like infection, suppuration and even sepsis. Pyrogen is also known as **'Homeopathic dynamic antiseptic'** because it acts effectively in septic fever especially puerperal. Post-operatively, Pyrogen would help to treat secondary infection; and septicemia developed after abortion. Great pain, and offensiveness of discharges (vomiting, diarrhea, pus, etc) with intense restlessness are marked indication of Pyrogen. Most characteristic feature of this remedy is the disparity between the pulse rate and the temperature. For instance, the pulse is 60 though there is high fever or it can be vice-versa. Pyrogen can be given in 30C or higher dose, but should not be repeated frequently.

  Rubrics from Synthesis Repertory 8.1 edition:

  Generals – Septicemia – ailments from

  General – Pulse – discordant with temperature

The above 11 remedies cover most of the pre and post-operative surgical injuries, but there can be different remedies than those mentioned above. Homeopathic remedies will act only if the similimum is achieved and symptoms are matched. Don't just throw the group of medicines on the patients. Observe, understand and find the similimum correctly to cure any patients.

IV. Conclusion

- Pre-operative and post-operative surgical wounds are very common. Pre-operative wounds or injury mainly includes mental injuries like anxiety, fear, restlessness, sleeplessness, etc. and physical complaints like diarrhea, fever and vomiting before the surgical process.

- Post-operative surgical wound includes, excessive bleeding, bruises, secondary infection from the incised wound, sepsis, fever, etc.

- Homeopathic remedies are effective in treating both pre and post-operative injuries or wounds. However remedy should match with the patient's symptoms appropriately.

Chapter 10: Head Injury / Brain Injury

I.   Introduction

Head injury is very commonly seen in children. Head injury is also called as brain injury or traumatic brain injury. Trauma either due to fall, or any mechanical force cause an injury to the brain is usually referred as **'brain injury' or 'traumatic brain injury'**. Head injury can be a small bump over the head due to fall or it can be severe brain injury affecting the life of a person.

Traumatic brain injury is very different than soft tissue injuries, or injuries to other body parts. In brain injury, one moment a person is fine while another moment life has abruptly changed. Injury to brain do not heal like other injuries and it has serious consequences than injuries to other body part. Some of the consequences are mental dysfunction, seizures, or even death. Hence it is important to treat it immediately and cautiously with continues monitoring of the vitals.

II.   Types and Causes of head injury

Traumatic brain injury are mainly cause either due to violent blow or blunt force over the head causing contusion, or sharp object penetrating the skull such as bullet causing deep damage to the brain. Head injury can lead to concussion to the brain where a person may feel little dizzy with a loss of vision and balance for a while.

A mild trauma to brain can cause mild or temporary dysfunction of the brain cells, while the severe brain trauma can result in bleeding due to torn tissues, bruising, and ultimately leading to long term complications or death.

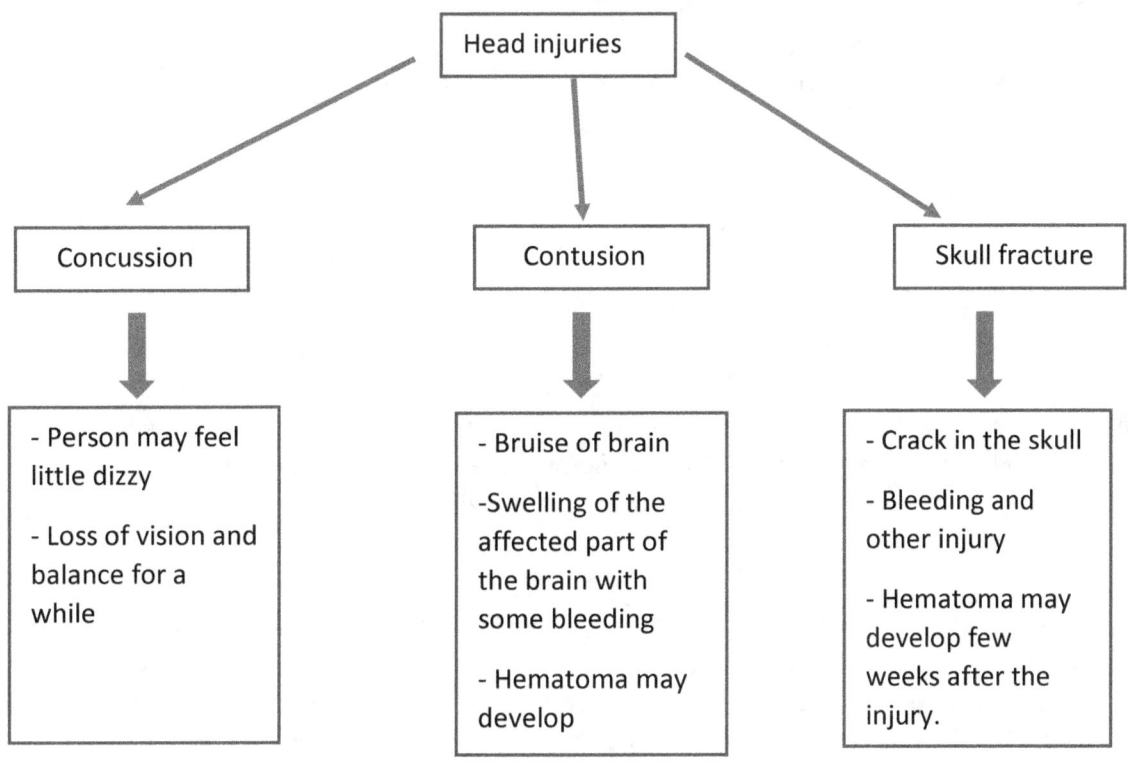

Types of head injuries, sign and symptoms

Mild injury to brain usually produces following symptoms:[15,16]

1) Brain injury is considered as mild if loss of consciousness and /or confusion and disorientation is shorter than 30 minutes.
2) Physical symptoms like nausea, vomiting, fatigue, and drowsiness.
3) Cognitive problems like headache, lack of memory, difficulty thinking, attention deficit and mood swings.
4) Sensory problems like blurring of vision, ringing in the ears, change in the taste and lack of ability to smell. Sensitive to light and sound.
5) Most of the time MRI/ Cat scans are normal.
6) Often it is an overlooked injury.

Severe injury to brain produces following symptoms:[15,16]

1) Severe brain injury is associated with loss of consciousness for more than 30 minutes
2) Memory loss for more than 24 hours
3) Persistent headache and vomiting
4) Loss of coordination, numbness or weakness of fingers or toes.
5) Convulsions , inability to awaken from sleep

6) Dilatation of pupils of eyes
7) Clear fluids draining from eyes and ears.
8) Cognitive problems like slurred speech, aggressive or unusual behavior, profound confusion and comatose condition.

III. Treatment for head injuries

Any brain injury, either mild or severe, requires immediate medical attention and treatment. Homeopathy works well mainly in case of mild injury to the brain. It does not mean homeopathy does not yield good result for severe brain injuries. In case of severe brain injuries it is important to first provide an emergency treatment to the patient, once the patient recovers homeopathic management would be useful to recover the patient from the trauma. Some of the research studies shows the effectiveness of homeopathic treatment for mild traumatic brain injury.[17]

Selection of homeopathic remedies are based upon the individualization and totality of symptoms (symptoms similarity). This approach will not only help to manage the head injury symptoms but will also achieve the complete state of health. A qualified homeopath will address the underlying cause if head injury and regain the disturbed vital force and susceptibility through the correct remedy.

i. Common homeopathic remedies for head injury

Following are some of the common homeopathic remedies useful in head injuries:

- **Arnica**

  Arnica is the most common remedy and should be the first remedy to think of in head injuries. Arnica is well known to rapidly heal mechanical and blunt injuries.[18] As described in previous chapters, Arnica is useful when there is sore and bruised feeling at physical and/or mental level. Here we will consider the feeling at physical level only. Arnica is not only useful for superficial bruises but also useful in severe brain injuries too.

  Arnica can be prescribed when a child falls from bed over the head or hits the wall with a bump over the head. It will heal the bruises and relieve the pain immediately. Along with Arnica, externally, compress the affected part with ice pack so that it does not swell further.

  Arnica works well in concussion of brain, even in compression of brain due to skull fracture or effusion of blood in the cranial cavity or in case of hematoma, however these severe brain injuries demand surgery in order to obtain immediate relief and permanent relief. Personally I have not seen complete cure from Arnica in serious brain injuries.

Dose: Depending on the acuteness of the case, repeat the dose. If the pain and bruises are severe repeat Arnica 30C or 200C, 4-5 times a day until the symptoms subsides.

Rubrics from Synthesis repertory 8.1:

Generals – Convulsions – brain – commotion of the ; from

Generals – Convulsions – injuries from – head of

Head – injuries of head, after

Head – Pain – injuries, mechanical

Head – Concussion of brain

- **Cicuta**
When the well-known remedy fails to act, the time comes to think out of the box. Cicuta is one of the remedy to think of in head injury. **Cicuta is mainly indicated when the functioning of brain is paralyzed with complete loss of consciousness.** Person gets convulsions, or epilepsy from concussion of brain. The convulsions of Cicuta are the most violent and are often accompanied by bizarre distortions. There is a state of unconsciousness or a dull dream like state following convulsion continuing for a long period of time, even a whole day.

After head injury, a person goes into mental retardation and frequent convulsions. During convulsions, frightful contortions will be seen in such patients, like head drawn backward, biting of tongue, strabismus (crossed eyes).

Dose: Cicuta can be given in 30C potency with less frequent repetition.

Rubrics from Synthesis repertory 8.1 edition:

Mind – unconsciousness – concussion of brain, from

Generals – Convulsions – brain – commotion of the; from

Generals – Convulsions – consciousness without

Generals – Convulsions – aura, stomach in

Generals – Convulsions – injuries from – head of

Generals – Convulsions – opisthotonos with

Head – Concussion of brain

Head – Pain – injuries, mechanical

Head – injuries of head, after

- **Hypericum**

As discussed in the previous chapters, Hypericum is a great remedy for injuries to the nerves and spine. Hypericum can be thought for fractured skull following head injury resulting in convulsions and loss of memory. Hypericum is usually followed by Arnica. [4]

Dose: For acute problems, prescribe Hypericum 30C or 200C pills for 3-4 times a day.

Rubrics from Synthesis Repertory 8.1 edition:

Mind – unconsciousness – concussion of brain, from

Generals – Convulsions – injuries from – head of

Generals – Convulsions – tetanic rigidity, traumatic

Generals – Convulsions – brain – commotion of the; from

Head – injuries of head, after

Head – Pain – injuries, mechanical

- **Natrum sulphuricum**

It is a deep acting remedy and widely used as a specific remedy for head injury. This remedy acts well when mental symptoms are taken into consideration along with physical complaints. Natrum Sulphuricum is one of the most important remedy in suicidal patients from, whether from grief, or head injury or other organic causes. Hence suicidality or suicidal thoughts after head injury is an indication of this remedy. Generally Natrum Sulphuricum patients are very responsible people, and have great sensitivity like weeps from hearing music.

Natrum Sulphuricum is primarily useful in after effects of concussions. Hence this remedy is more effective in mild brain injury and to some extent for severe brain injury. **Confusion, mental dullness, depression and convulsions after head injury are one of the important aspect of this remedy.** For old history of head injury Natrum Sulphuricum works to a great extent.

Headache with photophobia after head injury is also indicative of Natrum Sulphuricum.
Natrum Sulphuricum can be administered orally in the form of pills in 30c dose 2-3 times a day.

Rubrics from Synthesis Repertory 8.1 edition:

Mind – Suicidal thoughts – restrains himself because of his duties to his family

Mind – unconsciousness – concussion of brain, from

Mind – Suicidal – injury to head or brain; from

Head – Pain – injuries, mechanical, after

Head – injuries of head, after

- **Helleborus**
Helleborus is indicated when after injuries and blow to head, especially when there is stupefaction of brain and mind is completely blank. Hahnemann described the state of stupefaction as ' where with sight unimpaired, nothing is seen very clearly,; with hearing perfectly sounds nothing is heard distinctly.' **Mental dullness and poor concentration is marked.**

It works well in head injury when a person will answer slowly with great effort; his memory becomes so weak that he can hardly remember what was said to him; goes into depression with suicidal tendency.

Dose: Helleborus can be taken in 30 C potency orally 2-3 times a day. Depending on the acuteness of the complaint, it should be prescribed. Personally I have seen only one dose of Helleborus 30C working for significant amount of time. Usually frequent doses are not required.

Rubrics from Synthesis Repertory 8.1 edition:

Mind – Stupefaction – injury to head after

Mind – Stupefaction – headache during

Mind – Suicidal – thoughts – mental power, from despair about loss of.

- **Hyoscyamus Niger**
Hyoscyamus patient experiences excitation of nervous system after head injury or concussion to brain. **Excitation of nervous system is in the form of delirium, mania with rage, restlessness, cursing and or exhibition of other inappropriate behavior.**

Gestures, chore-like; restless fingers; muttering; etc, shows the delirium stage of hyoscyamus. Hyoscyamus is indicated if patient develops convulsions, with excitation of nervous system.

Lascivious mania is common aspect of Hyoscyamus where he/she uncovers the whole body, and sings obscene songs. Mania with ridiculous gestures. Convulsive jerks of single muscles, or sets of muscle with long lasting muscle spasms.

Vision gets affected too. Dimness of vision; object looks red as fire, or too large or appear smaller. Speech is difficult and confused. Paralysis of tongue. All these effects on head, vision and speech are after effects of head injury and concussion to brain.

Dose: Hyoscyamus can be prescribed orally in 30c or 200c potency, three times a day.

Rubrics from Synthesis Repertory 8.1 edition:

Mind – Mania – lascivious

Mind – Mania – rage with

Generals – Convulsions – epileptic, accompanied by spasms; violent

Generals – Convulsions – fright, from

Head – injuries of head, after

- **Cuprum Metallicum**
  Cuprum Metallicum is another remedy useful in after effects of head injury, however this remedy is occassionally used for head injuries. Cuprum is specific remedy for seizures and epilepsy after concussion of brain.

  Cramps and spasms with epilepsy which develops after head injury is the striking indication of Cuprum Metallicum.
  Delirium is of violent character where the patient bites; and loquacious delirium. Convulsion with blueness of face and lips, and froth at mouth. The convulsion is followed by deep sleep.

  According to Vithoulkas, Cuprum metallicum patients has intense emotions or impulses which are strongly suppressed. In order to maintain control over strong emotions, patient rigidly closes down every expression. Hence this suppression comes out in the form of spasms and convulsions. Even though it seems head injury is the main cause for convulsions, deeper case taking will help you understand the patient clearly. Hence Cuprum Metallicum may not be the first remedy of indication in head injury.

  Dose: Cuprum metallicum can be given in 30c pills for 1-2 times a day.

  Rubrics from Synthesis Repertory 8.1 edition:

  Generals – Convulsions – injuries from – head of the

  Generals – Convulsions – falling, with

  Generals – Convulsions – consciousness with

- **Stramonium**

  Head injury causes violent jerks in Stramonium patients. Behavior of Stramonium patient is very similar to Hyoscyamus, only difference is the degree of violence and fear of violence.

  Stramonium is highly violent than Hyoscyamus. The rage is uncontrollable and impulsive and comes in an outburst as convulsion. These patients are equally fearful too.

  Stramonium can be wisely used in severe brain injury. It is may not be your first choice of remedy in head injury. However it can be the best remedy to complete the cure.

  Dose: Stramonium can be given orally in 30 C potency, 1-2 times a day.

  Rubrics from Synthesis Repertory 8.1 edition:

  Mind – violent – deeds of violence; rage leading to

  Generals – Convulsions – tetanic rigidity, traumatic

  Generals – Convulsions – tetanic rigidity, trismus with

  Generals – Convulsions – falling, with

  Generals – Convulsions – consciousness with

IV. Conclusion

- Head injury is also referred as brain injury or traumatic brain injury. Trauma due to fall, or any mechanical force cause injuries to the brain.

- The brain injury is mainly cause either due to violent blow or blunt force over the head or sharp object penetrating the skull. Such violent trauma leads to contusion, concussion to brain or fracture of skull. Brain injuries are commonly seen in athletes like football players.

- Mild and severe brain injuries requires immediate medical treatment to avoid further consequences.

- Homeopathic remedies work very effectively in mild head injury. In severe kind of head injury, homeopathic remedies may or may not work effectively.

V.   References

14. *Traumatic brain injury*. (2014, May 15). Retrieved from Mayoclinic:
    http://www.mayoclinic.org/diseases-conditions/traumatic-brain-injury/basics/symptoms/con-20029302

15. *Traumatic brain injury.com*. (n.d.). Retrieved from
    http://www.traumaticbraininjury.com/understanding-tbi/what-are-the-effects-of-tbi/

16. Chapman EH, W. R. (1999 Dec). Homeopathic treatment of mild traumatic brain injury: A randomized, double-blind, placebo-controlled clinical trial. *J Head Trauma Rehabil.*, 521-42.